T0159961

The Upside of Being Down

the UPSIDE of BEING DOWN

of

the LIFE *of a* TEEN *with* ANOREXIA

Carolina Mejía Rodríguez

NEW YORK

LONDON • NASHVILLE • MELBOURNE • VANCOUVER

The Upside of Being Down

The Life of a Teen with Anorexia

Published in New York, New York, by Morgan James Publishing. Morgan James is a trademark of Morgan James, LLC. www.MorganJamesPublishing.com

ISBN 9781642797312 paperback
ISBN 9781642797329 eBook
Library of Congress Control Number: 2019946614

Cover Design by:
Rachel Lopez
www.r2cdesign.com

Interior Design by:
Christopher Kirk
www.GFSstudio.com

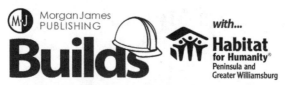

Morgan James is a proud partner of Habitat for Humanity Peninsula and Greater Williamsburg. Partners in building since 2006.

Get involved today! Visit
MorganJamesPublishing.com/giving-back

For Mamá, Papá, and Andres

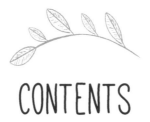

CONTENTS

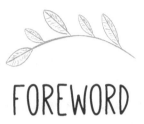

FOREWORD

This is a raw, gritty personal story of an exceptional young woman's brave journey through her illness and into recovery. I am grateful that Carolina shared her book with me and am honored that she asked me to contribute.

In the course of my medical training, I studied many erudite, scientific tomes to understand more about eating disorders to treat my patients effectively. Yet I have learned far more about the internal mental struggles of a patient and the despair her family might go through from reading this book.

When I first met her, Carolina was a very ill, underweight, depressed, and worried little girl. She had been sick for a couple of years and seen by quite a few doctors and therapists, all of whom had helped her in one way or another. She was still struggling, though. Her verbatim quote in my clinical notes from that first consult reads, "Oppressed by the voice in her head."

> She presented with classic diagnostic criteria of anorexia nervosa (DSM-5*):
> - Refusal to eat leading to significantly low body weight
> - Intense fear of gaining weight (she told me "thinner is better")
> - Persistent exercising that interfered with weight gain
> - Body image distortion
> - Low body mass index

Carolina writes accurately that anorexia nervosa is a "complex illness that encompasses much more than the refusal to eat." Many underlying biopsychosocial factors, unique to each individual, may contribute to falling ill. Her parents were recommended to start Family-Based Treatment (FBT), which has consistently been shown to have the highest success rate for anorexia nervosa treatment.**

FBT is a commitment not to be taken lightly because it requires much effort and time from all involved. Mom and Dad shouldered these responsibilities. Sook Ming (my best family therapist colleague) and I were so impressed at their first family meal when Adriana set the table with colorful place settings, letting us know she took this very seriously. We watched as Carlos took valuable time off from his busy work travel schedule so that he could *be there* at home and for therapy. And Andres came to every session to cheer up his sister. Most of all, we saw Carolina herself fighting against the negative voice in her head every step of the way. Successfully.

At our most recent consultation, the frightened little girl had grown up into a healthy, beautiful, and insightful young woman.

As mental health practitioners, we know FBT works and are very familiar with the psychotherapeutic techniques we trained in. Through this recovery journey of Carolina and her family, I learned another important lesson: love is the one driving force behind why and how a family helps their child to get well.

Privileged to be Carolina's doctor,
Dr. Lee Ee-Lian
Better Life Clinic Pte Ltd
10 Sinaran Drive #08-17/30, Novena Medical Centre,
Singapore 307506
Tel: +65-6-250 8077
email: clinic@better-life.sg www.better-life.sg

*Diagnostic and Statistical Manual of Mental Disorders (Fifth Edition)
**J Lock, D Le Grange, W. S. Agras, & C. Dare. Treatment Manual for Anorexia Nervosa: A Family-Based Approach

ACKNOWLEDGMENTS

What a journey this has been. So many people have inspired me to write this book. First of all, thank you to Morgan James publishing who has believed in my vision and helped me deliver this story to readers. Thank you to my great editor, Angie Kiesling, for opening your mind and accepting my book with its flaws, making it so much better. Thank you to the amazing teachers who helped me survive my middle school years. Thank you, Traci Massey, Paul Booth, and Ana Srepel; you are all inspiring individuals who have made a great impact on my world and that of my classmates. You will always be my teachers, for the lessons you taught me will forever evolve and accompany me through my adventures.

To Katrina Gillen, if our friendship has survived middle school, transcontinental moves, and crazy time zones, it will survive anything. Thank you to Victoria Carrillo, a true friend. You accepted me and supported me even though my situation was hard to understand—all the love and respect for my extended family.

Thank you to all the people who have been there for me. To my mentors and inspirations, thank you to the authors of the books that gave me comfort when I could find none.

If it weren't for my brother, I would not be here today. He might be obsessed with Marvel Superheroes, but he doesn't realize that the greatest hero stares at him from the mirror. He has been the most supportive and strong little brother anyone could ever ask for.

Thank you to my aunt, my rock, Tia. Ever since I made the phone call to tell you about my eating disorder, you stood next to me against the strong winds. Your calls and messages always brightened my day. Words cannot express what you did for my family and me. Thank you for taking care of my mom and helping her get out of her depression; you have been our lifeline.

Thank you to my cousin Mai, who I consider more of a big sister. You have been a vital part of this process, and without you I would still be hiding beneath the eating disorder. You have been and always will be an inspiration, and I aspire to be as kind and dedicated as you when I grow up. God didn't give me a biological sister, but He did give me you.

To Tatiana, the person who changed my view on the eating disorder. You were the one who helped me realize that recovery was in my hands all along. You changed my life forever.

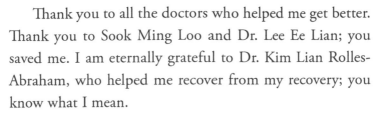

Thank you to all the doctors who helped me get better. Thank you to Sook Ming Loo and Dr. Lee Ee Lian; you saved me. I am eternally grateful to Dr. Kim Lian Rolles-Abraham, who helped me recover from my recovery; you know what I mean.

To my father, my inspiration, my hero. I admire your strength and your willingness to grow as a person. Your lessons will stay with me forever. You have given me the world, and one day I will give you the stars. Be strong, be happy.

Finally, to the person who kept me alive. My mom, my other half, my best friend. We have fought, cried, and laughed together. Thank you for giving me the best gift I will ever receive, your trust. There aren't enough words in our language for me to truly express my love for you. Without your support and understanding, I would not be here.

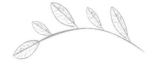

A NOTE FROM THE AUTHOR

This book documents my experience with anorexia nervosa, a complex illness that encompasses much more than the refusal to eat. Many details may be sensitive for certain readers, but the goal of this book is to help readers understand anorexia from the perspective of a teenager who experienced it firsthand. I was diagnosed when I was eleven, and at fourteen, I am finally leaving that hole of darkness.

It is important to understand that an eating disorder is not about vanity or wanting to look a certain way. That is only a component. Control is what it is truly is about. In my fourteen years of life, I have lived in five different countries because that is my family's lifestyle. I have never been able to control my life, the path set before me.

And while I like our life, I coped with this lack of control by controlling the only thing I truly could: what went in or out of my mouth. If I tried hard enough, I was able to control how my body looked and how I felt. Unfortunately, my need to control, amongst many other things, led to years of suffering from an eating disorder.

Everyone has different experiences with mental health and I am not comparing mine with others. This is simply my story and one that has been hard for me to open up about. This book isn't meant to be perfect; it's meant to be real.

1

COLOMBIA: GROWING PAINS

Kids can be cruel. When you are in third grade, your school is your oyster, and just like Bilbo Baggins in *The Hobbit,* you are on a quest. The quest is not to reclaim Lonely Mountain and recuperate riches from a dragon. Instead, most are on a quest to be liked. I was no different.

Walking down the stairs of my third school (I had been born in Mexico, then moved to the United States, and at the time I was living in Bogotá, Colombia), I saw two girls whispering and laughing. I stealthily approached them, for curiosity got the best of me. The short brunette started talking about a girl in our grade and how she was so weird and dumb. The other one, following the lead, laughed, even though you could see that she didn't understand what was so funny. Then, the brunette pressed her lips into a straight line and furrowed her brows, turning the light conversation into a serious matter.

"So," she asked, "from one being the worst to ten being the best, how much would you rate her?" She stuck her arm out and pointed at the girl she had previously insulted with words too graphic and insulting to mention.

Looking back, I would not think it possible for eight-year-olds to know how to use such phrases. The other girl's cheeks turned red like a tomato, and her eyes started moving around, looking at the faces of the other girls who had joined in. At that moment, the girl knew this wasn't a question but a test of her loyalty to the brunette.

"Um," she stammered as she licked her lips, turning to see if anyone would come to help her. After all, the girl they were talking about was pretty nice. She had her tough moments and could have temper swings, but, all in all, she was sweet and willing to help anyone who needed it. Nevertheless, this whole awkward exchange was happening, and it was a problem.

Daily, kids—including me—are peer pressured into saying and doing things they would never say or do on their own. Finally, the conflicted girl announced, "I guess I would rate her a four?" She answered in a way that made it seem more like a question than a statement.

"Good, that means you are in the club!"

That is how I also ended up being part of a club that recruited more and more kids to hate an innocent girl. The pressure crushed me as if I were diving into the deepest part

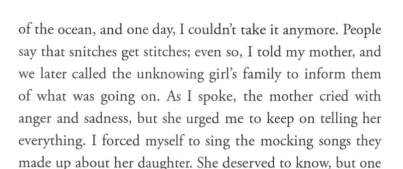

of the ocean, and one day, I couldn't take it anymore. People say that snitches get stitches; even so, I told my mother, and we later called the unknowing girl's family to inform them of what was going on. As I spoke, the mother cried with anger and sadness, but she urged me to keep on telling her everything. I forced myself to sing the mocking songs they made up about her daughter. She deserved to know, but one way or another, word got out, and the whole thing reversed. I ended up being the wounded soldier.

Everyone stopped talking to me. I tried to coax acceptance from classmates, but no one budged. The hatred emitted from my peers burned my skin. All my past efforts of laughing when I didn't think the joke was funny, saying things I didn't want to say, and doing things I didn't want to do failed—all because I dared to tell an adult about it. I was surrounded by deafening silence as the school year continued.

I slowly put on my one-piece bathing suit, the beautiful present my mother had bought me on one of her recent trips. It was white with a thousand blue flowers and a ruffled skirt just below my belly button. I tied my hair in a perfect bun, making sure no hair was out of place. After all, it was a pool playdate, and for a nine-year-old girl, nothing could be more important.

I had looked forward to that playdate for weeks. Finally, a girl in my grade enjoyed being with me! She didn't gossip or make fun of others, and she loved to read and laugh. After three long years of being untrue to myself, I was finding the courage to leave the group of kids who, for so long, had pressured me to be a person I wasn't.

During those years, the burdensome need for belonging had pulled me down like quicksand. Because of insecurity, I ended up being a loud and obnoxious girl who made stupid jokes to fit in, who said what people wanted to hear instead of what she really thought.

The popularity scale was clear and straightforward for me. Every day, I envisioned a plan to see who I had to befriend to climb the ladder because I knew that if I didn't, the snickers and comments from my classmates would be too much to bear. Yet, in the midst of all this, I started noticing things other children did not see at my age: I saw that all the girls did was pull each other down. I saw the fire of jealousy in the eyes of the girl who was supposed to be my best friend.

What I didn't notice, though, was the evil flare that was starting to grow in me. Instead of becoming the follower they wanted me to be, I became a self-deprecating girl who hated herself. Every day, I sank a little bit more. Happy to start freeing myself from the clutch of the "cliques," but unaware of the darkness simmering within, I put on that floral swimsuit. I thought my life was about was to change because I had finally found a true friend.

At some point, every girl starts paying attention to her body, its shape and size. It may be how her belly sticks out or how her legs rub together when she walks. After moving from the United States to Colombia at age six, I started looking at myself more. But my critique wasn't based on magazines or models; it was based on an image I had inside my head that represented beauty and self-acceptance. More

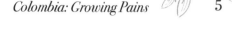

and more often, I pulled my shirt up and turned sideways in front of my mother to ask: "Am I fat? Do I have a belly? Am I bloated?"

The answer was always the same, "Yes, darling, you are a little bloated, but it's nothing to worry about; I assure you. Your body is preparing for all the changes you are going to go through. You are going to need a lot of energy so you can grow and thrive." In the moment, it was enough. I kept on eating candy and living the life of a normal kid. But as I grew, a nagging voice inside my head grew louder:

You are a burden to your parents.

You do nothing right.

You are fat and unlovable.

You don't deserve anything.

By the time I was nine, no matter how determined I was to ignore those terrible thoughts, they were consuming me. By worrying so much about being a burden to my parents, I ended up being one to myself.

On that promising Friday afternoon, wearing my floral swimsuit, I sprayed on some perfume, chose my best pair of sandals and the most beautiful pool towel I had, and headed out of my room to where my newfound best friend was waiting for me.

"Do you like the swimsuit?" I asked. "My mother bought it for me when she was in Spain!"

Her big hazel eyes looked at me as her hands fumbled in her lap. She tucked her golden locks carefully behind her ears. "Yeah," she answered, "you look good." That was the answer I wanted to hear. My nerves calmed, and I was once again able to control my fidgety toes.

"But," she continued, with a guilty look in her eyes, "there is something I really need to tell you." I turned to face her straight on, and my hands automatically crossed in front of my chest. My sweaty palms became rivers of water as I furtively tried to wipe them on my suit. My toes scraped against the surface of my sandals. I could feel my heart beating in my chest more quickly than it had before.

"Remember that sleepover I went to last week with all of the other girls in class?"

"Yeah, the birthday party I wasn't invited to," I answered.

"Yeah, I know," she said as she put her hands on her lap, taking a deep breath as if the words she was about to speak required great strength. I knew these words would likely do damage.

She continued, "Well, we were sitting there after dinner, and I don't remember exactly who started talking about it, but everyone in the house started talking about how fat you are."

Time slowed down. I looked at the tattered brown couch she was sitting on, and then my sight drifted toward the large window letting gray light in from outside, a dim grey that would later invade my soul. I took a few steps back to my room to look at my reflection in the mirror. The routine started once again. I first looked at myself sideways, then facing forward, next the other side, and finally, I turned around to see how I looked from the back.

"What did you say?" I asked, walking back into the living room. Unconsciously, I leaned on the wall beside me for support. At that moment, a confusing fog clouded my eyes, blurring my vision. Why was her comment so important? Yes, I knew I had started asking for uniforms that looked bigger on me so other kids wouldn't see my belly. Yes, I had tried to eat fewer carbs, but was it such a big deal?

Yes, it is a big deal.

"What did you say?" I repeated, an unknown fire burning in my chest. Was it anger? Was it shame? I had never been so aware of every feeling in my body. I noticed how my stomach churned as saliva flowed slowly down my throat; how my breaths became shorter, more frequent; and how I had an intense urge to move my hands and feet.

"Um," she stammered, "well, I didn't say anything. Don't worry; I didn't agree. I just listened. But, you know, since we are friends, I had to tell you. Please don't be mad at me."

"Oh, okay," I answered, convincing myself that I could trust her. "But, wait. Do you think I'm fat?" The question burst out as if a force stronger than me compelled me to ask it. At that very same moment, my mother walked into the living room.

"No!" my friend exclaimed. "Of course not!"

"Is everything okay?" my mother asked.

No! I wanted to yell. *Everything is not okay!*

"Yeah, mom, everything is fine. Don't worry," I quickly answered. Oblivious to the look on my mother's unconvinced face, I turned away. It is alarming how mothers always seem to know the truth, no matter how hard you try to act otherwise. I believe that my parents already knew there was a problem, but they were not quite sure how to go about solving it.

Nevertheless, I wasn't going to turn my insecurities into a giant snowball of predicaments for my parents. They already had enough to worry about. Over and over again, my parents were getting hints of the complex problems planting their roots in my brain, but I felt the need to protect them. I already worried them enough.

"Okay," Mom said, "head on over to the pool then."

I was still in a weird trance, but my friend seemed extremely relieved that the conversation was over. Her shoulders were relaxed as she rushed to the door and flashed a smile at me. I forced myself to chin up and smile. My insecurities and fear would just have to be dealt with later. The problem was, I did so too late.

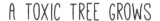

A TOXIC TREE GROWS

One day, the head cramps started. I was in my mom's room and decided to get a snack. I left the room, and after I had taken ten steps, I felt a cramp—not in my legs or in my abdomen but in my head.

I started yelping in pain. I grabbed on to the table beside me and squeezed my eyes shut. I felt the pain spread as tears streamed down my face. My mom came running out of the room and scooped me into her arms. I put my head on her chest and clutched the aching spot on my skull. I could feel my mother's heart beating as fast as a race car, and then suddenly, the pain stopped.

This repeated itself many times a day, and my parents finally decided to request medical tests. For hours and hours, I had to stay still with cables stuck to my head, breathing fast, breathing slow, blinking, yawning, smiling—everything the doctors told me to do. Every result said the same thing: nothing is wrong.

Nevertheless, no is not an answer for my parents; thus, they found a neurologist to perform more tests. When we got there, the doctor gave me a few simple coordination tasks. When the checkup was over, he handed my parents a slip of paper with instructions and dismissed us. Little did I know that the note told my parents to figure out what was going on at school because the head cramps were not normal. From that moment, a tree started to grow. The roots were a combination of insecurity, stress, and anxiety. As time passed, the tree grew, with millions of fears and worries disguised as leaves that would not let me lead a normal life. Who knew that trees and leaves could destroy you?

2

COLOMBIA: TWISTED FINGERS

We have all heard that those who love us are the ones most likely to hurt us, yet we never actually believe we are at risk. After all, they do love us. Right? In many households, sometimes a lion is waiting to attack the defenseless gazelle.

I was about to become the gazelle in my own home.

May was approaching, and after two hard years of waking up early for religion class, my first communion was only days away. Mine was not a strictly religious household. Nevertheless, I couldn't wait for the day to put on my white, puffy dress, walk down the church aisle, and receive holy communion for the first time. To be completely honest, I was also extremely excited about the party my parents were going to hold for me after the ceremony. Oh, all of the gifts!

My father's sister was going to give me my first cell phone, the highly revered iPhone 4.

The day went just as planned. I had my hair done; my wild curls were tamed and held in place by a flamboyant bow. In complete sincerity, the wafer and wine tasted horrible, but the happy time I had afterward seemed too good to be true.

After the festivities had passed and every visitor had left, my mother, her two sisters, and her mother went on a women-only trip to Europe. They were ecstatic with the idea since they had not done a trip like this in a long time. Unfortunately, my father had to travel for work as well, so my brother and I were left in Colombia with a family member who moved into our home to care for us.

One night, after getting ready for bed, we decided to watch TV together. The night was cold, and I remember the cozy lighting of our living room. Suddenly, our caretaker grunted and looked at me with fiery eyes. I looked up, pausing from making a bracelet, and waited to see if she had said something.

"Look what you did!" she exclaimed, pointing her long, thin fingers at our old TV.

"What did I do?" I asked, feeling a horrible pain in my stomach.

"You turned the TV off! How could you? You know I like that show!"

"I didn't turn it off; it just does that sometimes," I answered, worrying about her aggressive arms waving in the air, her face turning as red as fire. My brother, who was only four years old, cowered on the couch, moving as close to the edge as possible. Sometimes, when lightning strikes, the world seems to stop for a few moments, and that is precisely what happened that night.

"Go to your room!" she yelled. I was shocked by her outburst. Never before had I seen such hatred and anger in a person who was supposed to take care of me. I quickly skidded out of the living room, leaving my little brother behind. Instead of going to my own room, I ran to my parents' bedroom, hoping the storm would calm in the morning.

The next morning, she acted as if nothing had happened, so I decided to hide my fear and sadness. School was the usual routine, and by the end of the day, all I wanted to do was go back home and rest.

The bus rolled up in front of my apartment building. I stepped off and went home. As I opened the door, I left my backpack and went directly to my room; strangely, I heard a whimpering noise inside. I peeked through the door and saw her sobbing on the phone.

"I can't take it anymore!" she wailed. "I can't stay here with these children. Carolina is so cruel to me! I need to go back home!" I looked around to see if my little brother was near. I couldn't let him see this woman in such a state. I quickly whispered my greetings and went once again to my parents' room. After a few moments, I heard angry stomps getting closer. *Bang!* The door swung open, and she was standing in front of me.

"You ungrateful little girl! I am here to help your parents, and you don't even have the manners to say hello when you come home?" she yelled, pointing her fingers at my face. Those were the fingers that used to tickle me silly. Those were the fingers that used to hug me tight. Those were the fingers of my loving relative, but the woman I had come to know wasn't the person I thought she was.

"I swear I did say hello. I just saw you talking on the phone, so I didn't want to interrupt," I said, starting to lose my patience.

"Do you think I am dumb? My ears are working perfectly well! I would have known if you had said hello!"

"But I did say it!" I retorted as all my poise slipped away.

"Don't you scream at me!" she said in such an aggressive voice that I was forced to move back. I curled up in a ball and waited until she left. Tears streamed down my face as I heard the last of her footsteps trail out of the door. Finally, she was gone. I had never thought I would be so glad to see a family member go.

Now it seemed to me that I wasn't safe at school *or* home. My mind was racing with internal interviewers, all flashing questions at me, demanding answers: *Is she screaming at my brother, too? Do I deserve this? What did I do wrong?* The questions seeped into my mind, creating even more confusion. The darkness that fell as the sun went to sleep made my soul quiver. At that moment, I just wanted my mom and dad. I cautiously climbed onto my parents' bed and hid under the covers. *Why isn't anyone helping me?*

The next morning, I woke with a startle. The phone was ringing, and my heart was racing, hoping it was my mom. I scrambled out of my fort and answered the phone. The door to the room was still closed as I quietly told my mom what had happened. She said that I should keep strong and she would be home in a few days. But my tears were too loud, and the monster in my house stormed into the room once again.

Snatching the phone out of my hands, she glared at me and started screaming into the phone, "I am not mistreating your daughter; she is being very difficult to deal with right now." I jumped out of bed, and as she closed the call, she chased me around the house, screaming about what a liar I was. With no place to hide, I locked myself in the bathroom. As if in a movie, I dramatically slid down the door and was covered in tears. I heard my brother's small steps outside of the door like a confused puppy, but I could do nothing for him. I was too vulnerable. Once I was ready for school, I rushed out the front door. Maybe today would be different.

After school, I got home and found the house so quiet, one could hear a pin drop. I believed that to be a good sign, so I proceeded to my parents' bedroom once again, but as I sat down and turned the TV on, the house started to shake. The tornado that was once part of my family charged into the room with our maid running behind her, pleading for her silence.

She raised her arms in a choking motion and told me in a threatening grumble, "No one is ever going to believe you. If you tell them what happened, they will all be on my side. You will be left alone. Your father will only believe me; he will never trust you again." Her voice shook, and I pictured everything she was saying. I saw an enormous brick wall that separated me from everyone else. An unusually sinister grin rested on her face as she looked down at me with disapproval.

Was she right? Tears seemed like a constant decoration on my face. *Would my tears run out?* As I stood up and shuffled my feet backward in an attempt to get away, she pulled out her phone. I could see that she was calling her own daughter.

"Tell her all of the things you have told me, ungrateful brat!" she yelled, shaking the phone as if to crush it with her anger.

"Please stop this!" the maid yelled as she put herself between me and the phone. I immediately saw the chance to escape and ran out of the room. A seed of guilt, fear, and distrust had just been planted, and I would have never imagined how big the poisonous weeds would grow.

I didn't have the strength to call my mother, and there was no chance I would tell my father about this, so I wrote down everything that had happened. My mother called me through FaceTime several times a day, frustrated by the distance between us and her inability to cut short her cruise.

"You know I would never have left you there with her if I had known this would happen," my mom said in a cautious voice.

"Yes, I know," I answered, "but I'm scared, Mamá. I don't want to be here with her. My brother is also having to listen to all of this. I don't think I can take it."

"Well," she answered, "your father is closer than I am, so we are going to have to tell him. He is the only one who can help you right now."

"He won't believe me," I whimpered. "He'll think I am just being rude and mean. Please, don't tell him! I'll wait until you come home." My mother quickly changed the topic, telling me how hard this trip had been on her. The past few months had been tough since my grandma's sister had just passed away, and everyone was somber. My mom told me about how she had a corner on the cruise where she would sit and cry, feeling impotence and anger for not being able to help me or mitigate my grandmother Coqui's loss. Guilt over ruining my mother's trip seemed to drown me, pulling every good thing out of my body.

Determined to make my mother feel better so she could enjoy her trip, I tried to make her laugh.

"Send me a picture of the corner," I said jokingly as she wiped her pixelated eyes and blew me a kiss. After I gathered the courage to tell my dad about the situation with my family member, he cut short his business trip and immediately came home. Everything was back to normal.

With my father in the house, the tornado started acting like the loving relative I used to know, but after seeing and experiencing such things, I could not completely forget. That same day he arrived, she went back to her home city, but things weren't resolved. On the contrary, the problem was just beginning. Every time she would call my dad, he would hand me the phone in an attempt to start a conversation between us once again. I tried to put on a smile, wanting my dad to be calm and happy. After all, he flew all the way from Peru just to get me out of this situation, even though he was with the CEO of the company he worked for.

He dropped everything and came to my rescue, so I couldn't disappoint him by showing the fear I had every time I spoke to her. My dad was trying to heal wounds on both sides, claiming that this family member was "not herself"; thus, I should be compassionate and forgiving. Despite my dad's efforts to restore our former relationship, I had experienced these family confrontations for the first time, and the bad parts were now too obvious to ignore. The incident was to stay with me for many years to come.

THOSE WHO LOVE YOU

Months and months passed, and the seeds of insecurity slowly and silently wrapped themselves around my health. On a hot July morning, our plane landed in Cartagena, Colombia, the only place in the world I can, indeed, call home. We collected our baggage and ran toward Coqui, hugging her until she beckoned us into the car.

Out of the window, I could see the waves crashing against the sand and people in their swimsuits relaxing, letting the sun burn off their worries. Cartagena is a beautiful city that is full of history, wonderful architecture, and awe-inspiring beaches. It is a city I never get tired of visiting. As we arrived at my grandmother's apartment, I saw a tall and robust figure opening his arms. Tico. I ran toward my grandfather and saw his bright smile. Immediately, I jumped into his arms, and he swung me around.

"Cosi, cuanto te extrañé!"

"I missed you, too!" I replied, giving him a kiss on his bald, shiny head.

"I have a surprise for you!" I said, pulling him into the bedroom where my grandmother had already found a place to sit down. I smiled and pulled my shirt up so that he could only see my belly. A look of confusion registered on their faces, but my pride did not falter.

"Remember last time, when you told me I should lose some weight?" I asked with a glint of pride in my eye. I turned sideways, "Look at my belly now! It's less big!" He laughed and shook his head.

"Oh, wow! You look better than ever, *me derrito*!" He always used this phrase when he saw me; it means, you make me melt. A smile of accomplishment was tattooed on my face. Finally, I had shown him I could be thinner.

Everything was great; life couldn't be better, except my pride over losing weight had planted a seedling in my mind. The garden of poisonous weeds was growing larger without anyone knowing. Yes, I had proven to my family that I could be thinner, I could fit in, but my efforts had also watered the seeds of insecurity.

A few months later, we moved from Colombia to Chile. Finally, after four dark years, I escaped from Bogotá—not the city itself but the situation I was in. The night I figured out that we were moving, I cried for about three minutes. I cried because I would be farther away from my family. I cried for fear of starting over. But that was it. After I shed a few tears, I started smiling as I realized I was leaving my horrible life behind. I now had the great opportunity of starting from scratch. Now I would most assuredly leave behind the darkness that entered my soul the day of the floral swimsuit. I was going to be a different person. I was going to be me.

Indeed, within the first few days of school, I met a group of new kids who ended up being my best friends until I left Chile. We all liked the same weird things and enjoyed playing and laughing. For the first time in years, I felt like I belonged. I had finally found friends who wouldn't betray me or hurt me. They would simply be there for me.

The first year in Chile was great. All of my family members adapted quickly to what was going to be our new home. The school had great facilities. It was the first time I attended a school with a swimming pool, open spaces with tall trees where you could study, and pizza Fridays. I made many friends and brought my social skills up to date after my experiences in Colombia. In complete honesty, nothing could have been better.

Fifth grade, stereotypically, is the year that defines childhood. It's a period of time in which you are innocent, energetic, and happy. Even so, one thing still bugged me. My mom had bought me a bright pink sweater to wear to school because in Chile, during winter, temperatures can go down to zero degrees Celsius. At first, I wore it with pride. My school attire consisted of my puffy sweater, school pants, and my Gryffindor scarf, which I wore to school every day. Slowly, I started realizing that the sweater was tight in all of the wrong places and that my belly stuck out. I had to do something about it.

Maybe it would be better if you didn't eat pizza on Fridays.

Eat some fruit for afternoon snack instead of having lunch.

I decided to take matters into my own hands and became more conscious about what I ate and when I ate it. After all, I was going to middle school in less than three months and could make my own decisions. That summer, my brother and I flew to Colombia while my parents took a solo trip to Palm Springs.

With my parents away, my grandma and my aunts were in charge of taking care of me. I convinced them to get me into tennis lessons every day. I didn't really like running or swimming, and I had to do a sport, so they enrolled me in tennis class. One day, I got coughing fits. The bags under my eyes grew, and I could feel gravity pulling down on me. One of my aunts and my grandma agreed I should stop going to tennis, but I convinced them that I was fine.

However, my grandma was not satisfied. She asked me why I was so sad, if I wanted to take any medicine, if I wanted to cuddle. All in all, she played the role of concerned grandma very well. Two weeks passed, and my parents flew to Colombia to pick us up to go back to Chile. Another of my aunts and my cousin would meet us in Chile because we were going to take a trip to the desert together.

We got on the plane and landed safely back home, but that night, I was ambushed by coughing fits once again. My mother immediately took me to the hospital, and the doctors informed me that I had pneumonia. My mother's face went blank, and she looked back at me in utter shock.

Pneumonia? I thought. *I'm feeling fine. I just have a cough. What about the trip? Can I exercise?* Questions raged in my head like grains of sand in a sandstorm.

The doctor put me on antibiotics, and I was bed bound for the next two weeks. While my family headed up to the mountains to ski, I did my make-up and watched movies, wondering why the timing of my illness had to be so bad.

My brother says I am the queen of manipulation. He doesn't understand how I manage to persuade my parents into either buying us a gift or taking us to the mall, but when the doctor said we should reconsider our trip to the desert, my argumentative powers bloomed in all their splendor. I had to convince my mom that I was completely fine and ready to go on the trip. I made music videos with my cousins to the soundtrack of *Grease* to show my mother that my lungs were capable of maintaining physical activity for an extended amount of time. Finally, my mom gave in and said that she would take me on the trip, but I had to check in with the doctor before going. I agreed to this compromise, and the very next day, we headed to the doctor's office.

He checked my height, my lungs, my heartbeat, and my weight. "Well," the doctor announced, "it seems as if you have lost two kilograms these past two weeks. This is normal, though. Losing appetite is common amongst patients with pneumonia."

I turned my head away from my mother and the doctor and smiled. I was ecstatic. Two kilograms! That was more than I had ever been able to lose by reducing my food and increasing my exercise routine. I felt this was my gateway to making my dreams come true. I finally had the opportunity to become the person I wanted to be.

The trip was extremely fun. We sand boarded in the Valley of Death, went up to the Tatio Geysers, and experienced the numbing temperature of minus fifteen degrees Celsius. It is definitely amongst the best trips I have ever taken. Plus, I was able to maintain my version of a good diet because my mom was too busy gossiping with her sister to pay attention to what I was or wasn't eating. It was the perfect situation. Life couldn't be better.

I believe every person has a reservoir of pain that is spread throughout their life. I figured I had already used up all of mine. In blunt terms, I was wrong.

3

CHILE: REBORN

One September afternoon, I got back from school in a jolly mood, ready to tell my mom everything about my day. I opened the door and walked around the house, calling, "Mom, I am home. Where are you?"

"Give me a second," a muffled voice seemed to respond from the bathroom.

Completely oblivious to the tone of my mother's voice, I ate a snack and started on my homework. After ten minutes or so, I knew something was wrong. My mom was always ready to embrace me and talk as soon as I came home. I went down the stairs and peered into the bathroom. The lights were off, and no one was there. I thought I had heard my mom's voice coming from down there, but proven wrong, I paced around the first floor of my house. I then went to the backyard and found my mother weeping on the phone.

"I tried to believe that I didn't see it coming," she bawled, "but we all knew this was going to happen eventually. All her anger and sadness had to come out sooner or later."

I had never seen my mom in such a state of despair. Suddenly, I became anxious. What was happening? How should I help? Did I do something wrong? I did not know what to do, so I simply ran toward her and hugged her, reasoning this was the only thing that helped me feel better. She stiffened at the touch of my arms wrapping around her. I knew then that I was not invited to hear the conversation she was having.

"I'll call you later," she said as she hung up the phone and wiped her tears.

Time stopped. The only thing my mom did was hug me and cry. I knew she must feel horrible and vulnerable, like a soldier in the middle of a battle they know is lost. We stayed in the same position for ten minutes. I wanted to speak but wasn't sure what to say. The devil on my shoulder told me tell her not to cry. After all, I hated seeing her like that. But the angel on my other shoulder told me to just wait and listen— as I often needed her to do for me. Fortunately, I let my trusty angel win, waiting while the bomb inside my mom exploded. Once all the tears drained from her face, she looked up from my shoulder, which was soaking wet with her tears.

"Please, Mom, I need to know what's going on. You haven't been yourself all week, and now I find you bawling on the phone. I have tried to ignore it, but I can't anymore, please."

"Your grandmother has dementia. She's losing her memory. Coqui can't even remember what she had for breakfast. We are losing her!" She was shaking her head, looking like a small child, confused and lost. "The woman who we once knew is fading away like a ship in the sea. The worst part is, we can't do anything about it."

I was thunderstruck. My hands trembled, my breath deepened, my eyesight blurred, and my toes started wiggling as they do when I am anxious. It wasn't only a change, it was an ending. She might forget me, our times together, our TV shows. No, she *will* forget me.

I was facing a dead end, and I needed the fog to clear. I knew I had to be strong and hold back the river that was welling up in my eyes. I saw my mom look at me, expecting me to make her feel better, but how? Everything she said was true. We couldn't reverse the disease, and these types of changes demand to be acknowledged. I could only imagine what my extended family was thinking at the moment. As far as I knew, a change this big was unexpected and very unwelcome.

"I don't know what to say." I felt my breath leave my body, and suddenly the dam broke. It was my turn to cry. We both let the river flow down our cheeks. We both let our tears rain down onto our clothes.

"There is something we can do. We can be with her, call her, drink out of the well until the last drop dries up. We have to love her and take care of her." I offered this encouragement to reassure her, but in moments of such angst, doing so can end up making things worse.

"Yes, you are right. I love you," she said, and, once again, we embraced. That conversation marked an ending, a painful one. Not all fairy tales have happy endings.

Change comes in different ways. A move, an illness, even something as simple as seasons; those are all types of changes. The only way to move on and grow is to embrace the change and make the most out of it.

In the aftermath of this event, I started noticing how our already strong family bond became firmer. It grew, just like Jack's beanstalk. It could reach higher heights and support greater weight. However, just like a Kevlar vest, this strength seemed to act like a cover—protective, yes, but hollow. I was about to find out just how empty it could feel.

I hoped the worst had passed. After all, what could be worse than being far away from a person you love who is deteriorating? Well, being close to a person you love who is rotting right in front of your eyes is actually worse.

That's the thing with Kevlar vests; they are strong and impenetrable on the outside, but they house a vulnerable being inside. I was raw and wounded by the news of my grandmother's health, but the world just continued on. Sometimes you wish it would stop for a moment because the pain you are feeling is so intense and real that you can't fathom how other people carry on living. The worst is, I had to carry on with mine.

WHERE THE WILD THINGS GO

October came in the blink of an eye, and CWW week was right around the corner. CWW stands for Classroom

Without Walls, a chance for the whole grade to get on a bus, leave the comfort of home, and stay in cabins with a bunch of stinking teenagers.

Maybe it's just me who detests these trips. What was it that I found so unsettling? Was it the uncertainty? Being far away from the Kevlar vest that was my family? I don't know, and I don't think I will every truly understand.

I had never gone on a CWW trip before, but I hated the thought of sleeping away from home. Previously, going on class trips was a pain because I never had friends who would understand if I felt homesick. However, I had finally found true friends who would be there for me. Thus, I decided to give it a chance. I was going on the trip, so we started buying the things I needed to go to Lagunillas: sweaters, flashlight, and hiking pants.

The day came closer and closer. I had a horrible feeling in my gut, just like the one you have when you are on a roller coaster. You are going up slowly, knowing something big and scary is coming but feeling vulnerable because you can't do anything about it.

The night before the trip, I was up in my room crying when I started feeling a horrible burning sensation in my chest, which traveled to my stomach, down to my legs, and shook every fiber of my being. I was losing control. That was the moment I broke. The glue that was holding my life together suddenly disappeared, leaving a storm of crazy emotions.

By pure instinct, my mother came rushing into my room to find me in a corner rocking back and forth, back and forth. The face she made once she saw me is one I will never forget. Her usual smile faded, and her shining eyes lost their spark.

She reached out for me, her mouth wide open. "Gorda! Qué te paso?" She ran toward me asking what was wrong, but I couldn't speak. My anxiety was not letting me breathe.

"Mami, siento que me voy a desmayar."

"You feel like you're going to faint because you are not breathing! Breath in . . . and out . . . in . . . and out."

"I can't do it!" I said as my eyes widened. My dad walked calmly into the room, whistling a song he sang as soon as he arrived home from work. Normally, my brother and I would race to the door to greet him (I won almost every time), but today was not a normal day. As he saw me lying in bed, with my mom beside me trying to calm me, his pace quickened and he swiftly embraced me.

"What is wrong?" he asked.

"No sé," my mom said. "I walked in and saw her rocking underneath her desk. She said she was getting dizzy." As if she had a moment of epiphany, she asked, "Is this about tomorrow's trip?"

"I don't want to go on the trip," I bawled. "I'm so scared."

My tears continued for minutes on end until my dad suddenly blurted out, "If this trip is making you feel like this, you don't have to go."

"But I do!" I said, contradicting my previous statement. "I'm not going to be the weird kid who doesn't go. On top of that, I wouldn't want to disappoint you guys again!"

"You have never, and will never, disappoint us," my mom said, sounding like a true parent. "We just don't want to see you get hurt!"

I rolled around in bed, pondering what my parents had said, but my stubbornness got the best of me. I had to go. I just had to.

The next day came, and the world continued, but I felt as if my heart was about to stop at any moment. Everything passed in a blur. Breakfast, car ride, school, and finally the dreaded goodbye. My mom and dad stood next to the bus, waving at me with big smiles on their faces as if looking at their grins would make me want to smile; of course, it didn't. The engine boomed as I sat next to my best friend. I waved one last time before leaving and then simply fell asleep.

It was about an hour and a half before we came to a stop. We got off the bus, and I ate one cereal bar, knowing I shouldn't eat the banana they were offering because bananas had too many calories. I couldn't afford more calories in my body because I would get fat and everyone would notice and . . . Thoughts can be destructive.

We did a bunch of activities up in the mountains of Chile where it was freezing cold. The grass was yellow, parched due to the dry climate, yet all around us there were green trees taller than anything I had ever seen. The air seemed to weigh less, my lungs capable of taking deeper breaths. We had escaped the pollution of Santiago, and if it weren't for a constant nagging in my chest, which I couldn't identify, I would have considered the scene beautiful.

We stayed in a small house made of stone. Before the trip, my mom told the teachers that my best friend and I should have a separate room from everybody else because I was extremely scared of the trip. My mother's wishes were my teachers' commands, and we got a tiny private room, which allowed me to escape if the situation became too overwhelming. (Plus, I could sleep with my stuffed animal without worrying about being laughed at.) Everything was fine. Well, everything was as good as it would get.

Then the dreaded moment came: time for dinner. I sat down, and in front of me was a big bowl of pasta. Shit. Pasta has a lot of calories and is all carbohydrates. A teacher conveniently sat beside me, so I ate, not wanting to call attention by not eating.

I left half the bowl of pasta and exited the dining room. I climbed up to the bunk I was sharing with my friend. I sat there and just sobbed. And sobbed. And sobbed. Mucus was dripping out of my nose, my eyes were burning, and my heart felt like it would stop. I pulled out my phone, which I had secretly brought on the trip, and started texting my mom. The only comfort I had at that moment was watching the three little bubbles pop on the screen to indicate that my parents were writing, that I wasn't alone, that they still cared. After about fifteen minutes, I was finally starting to control myself. Just as the teacher was walking in, I put away my phone.

"Are you okay?" she asked sweetly.

"Yeah. I'm fine." Those two words combined are the worst in the world. Yes, what I am about to say is a cliché, but it's true. Saying, "I'm fine," is not being polite; it is lying. It is denying help when you really need it, but that's never going to change. Those two words are inscribed in our brains like a code; it's just what we are programmed to say.

The next day was the hike. We set out early in the morning after I ate about two spoonfuls of granola; after all, granola has nuts, and nuts have fat, and fat is bad. We hiked through muddy trails and sloped hills, going farther and farther. Every moment, I would tire more, but I would not stop. I needed to burn the calories I gained from breakfast. My feet were covered in mud and my hands drenched in sweat, but the mountain kept going. Finally, after about three hours, we reached the peak, and our reward was lunch. They gave us a sandwich and an orange. I convinced myself that I didn't like sandwiches, so I simply ate half an orange and a granola bar.

That same night, we had a campfire. It was one of the most beautiful things I have ever seen. We laid on the bare ground and looked at the sky. Never had I seen the stars so clearly in my life; no lights hid the stars and no noises distracted me. The guide had a green laser, which he used to point at the balls of gas floating in the air.

"This," he said, "is the bear constellation, and that over there, that is Jupiter."

"What is that red thing parallel to Jupiter?" a kid asked, breaking the comfortable silence.

"That's Mars. See, kids? If you simply stop, breathe, and observe, so many things come into focus. Had you ever noticed that you could actually see other planets from

Earth? Probably not. Sometimes, you must drop everything and just see."

I had never been surrounded by sixth graders who were content in complete silence. Something in the night sky made us reflect, made us open our eyes. It was an experience everyone needed, something I *really* needed.

Later, I slid into the bunk bed and put on my head flashlight. Under the blankets, I read the only book that really made me feel at home, a book that gave me peace: *Harry Potter and the Sorcerer's Stone.* Immediately I felt as if I were home, snuggling in my own bed, simply reading.

When the trip finally ended, we got on the bus to go back home. I got out the of the bus and scanned the crowd to find my mom. She was on her way with my brother. I pushed everyone out of the way and hugged my mom and brother as hard as I could. As soon as I pulled back, my mother held both of my arms to examine me.

"Oh, Lord," she said, tears welling up in her eyes. "You are so skinny. You lost so much weight." I fidgeted and simply told her that the food was really bad and that I survived on granola bars. As I fed my mother the white lie, I couldn't help noticing the rattling sound of the leaves on the trees of my mind.

We got in the car with my best friend so we could drop her off at her house. When I got home, I showered and left that smoking, ugly, treacherous cabin behind.

I continued my routine, jogging five times a week, sometimes with my dad, sometimes alone. I couldn't help but go back to the comment my mom made as soon as she received me from the camping trip: "You are so skinny." This was a phrase I had never heard before, and I liked it.

Maybe if you reduce your food, you can be even thinner.

Prettier.

More acceptable.

That very week, my parents held a dinner at our house with some of our closest friends. It was as if my mom wanted to test me, to see if I would eat. Every second of every day, I felt as if someone were out to get me, as if I was hiding something. I can't quite explain the feeling fully, but it was a sort of paranoia that followed me everywhere. The dinner consisted of traditional Chilean choripan (a type of hot dog but made with baguettes and chorizo) and a variety of other carbohydrates.

Chorizo is very fatty, isn't it?

The bread has way too many calories.

Control yourself or you will never get thinner.

I calmly headed up to my room, deliberately avoiding the food and anyone with food, for fear that they would offer me some. But as I was about to go up the stairs, my mother pulled me by my arm.

"Aren't you going to eat anything?" she asked.

"I'm not really hungry," I said, convincing myself that what I was saying was true. Honesty in my family is a big deal. My parents have always expressed the importance of being honest, and we have cultivated a relationship in which I never lie to them, and they never lie to me.

Am I lying?

No.

I was about to continue on my way as one of the guests approached me and grabbed my waist. I could immediately feel each of her fingers on my ribs. I flinched. I had stopped letting people touch or hug me, something which really bothered my mom. As Latinos, our culture is all about expressing your love through hugs and kisses and, well, food—but that's another issue.

"Uy, Caro! What happened? You have lost so much weight!" the guest remarked. I looked up at my mom, her sweet, calm face now turned into a mask. She was still smiling, but it wasn't genuine. Her smile was the saddest thing I had ever seen.

"Yes," my mom responded. "She has been exercising quite a lot, cutting down the amount of food she eats."

"I see," the guest said, mimicking my mom's fake smile.

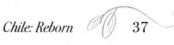

The tone of her voice made me think her remarks were not compliments but judgments. Nevertheless, she said "thin" in her sentence—now the most prized word in my vocabulary.

4

CHILE: LEAVES DON'T ONLY FALL IN AUTUMN

Halloween came, and the chilly air filled our surroundings, even though spring was supposed to be right around the corner. It was my second Halloween in Chile, and this time I had everything organized for it to be an amazing day. First, I would go to a party at the United States Embassy with my best friend. Then I would go home, change into my new costume, and go trick or treating around the condominium. This was every eleven-year-old's dream.

Everything was perfect. We had the time of our lives during the embassy event, getting scared by workers and receiving American candies, but the best part was simply that I had a friend who finally invited me to do something with her.

At the end of the event, I sorted through my candy to see which I would give to my brother, which I would save for my mom, and which I would give away. No way would I ingest those greasy, fatty, sugary pieces of food—not now that I was finally losing weight.

As I opened the front door to my house in my brightly colored witch costume, I called out for my mother. I wanted to show her all of the candy, but once again, she didn't receive me with her usual, happy embrace.

"Come," she stretched out her arms, "we need to talk." I saw her survey my legs, which were covered in colorful striped leggings. She took me to her room, and I dumped all of the candies on her bed.

"Look!" I exclaimed, grabbing a Reese's peanut butter cup and shoving it in her hand. "Your favorite! I grabbed it as soon as I saw it because I know they don't sell them here."

She smiled sadly and closed her grip on the chocolate.

"They were once your favorite, too." As tears gleamed in her eyes, looking like twinkling stars, she kept on talking, " I know how important your weight is to you." The stars were now exploding and flowing down her flawless face.

She continued, "But you are so, so thin. It's worrying me. Dad and I both agree that you aren't eating enough. A cheese sandwich at night isn't enough for you. Neither is the small portion of cereal you eat for breakfast. We think you need to go to a nutritionist and maybe even a psychologist. Remember the pictures of the girls I showed you online? The girls who looked like walking skeletons? I'm worried you'll start looking like them, and I don't want you to get sick."

It was true; she did warn me. Every day she showed me a picture of an anorexic girl with a sad and droopy face with a frown that stuck out more than the bones in her body. I couldn't help but shiver.

"I won't get sick, Mom!" I retorted. "Please don't send me to a doctor! I'm okay. I swear I am okay. Look, what if I eat this chocolate? If I eat it, you won't take me to the nutritionist, okay?" I looked into her eyes, but the only response I got was her endless tears that resembled a waterfall.

"Look, Mom! I'm eating it." I turned the small orange packaging in my hand and started unwrapping the peanut butter cup, the strong chocolate scent piercing my nose.

Don't do it. You'll get fat.

But then she won't take you to the doctor.

Eat it quickly and get it over with. You are not crazy; you don't need a doctor. Plus, you won't become like those skeletons with flesh. You know that won't happen.

I turned it around in my hand, letting the chocolate slowly melt in my trembling palm. My head cramped up, contracting from all of the stress and pressure the thought of eating the chocolate created. I opened my mouth and squinted my eyes as if I were being forced to eat a deadly poison. Forcing my arm to move, I stuck the Reese's peanut butter cup into my mouth. I could feel the calories transforming into fat, clinging to my belly, legs, and arms. My throat ached with the unbearable sweetness of the milk chocolate that melted in my mouth, just like my composure melted in my head.

Heavy sobs exploded out of me like an unexpected bomb. Tears came more fiercely than they ever had before, covering the sheets on the bed and drowning my happiness and calmness. More seeds were being watered and new leaves were about to appear on the tangled branches in my mind.

Days passed, and like a lion in a cage, I became desperate and agitated. My mother and father had confirmed I was going to go to a doctor. They promised me it was simply a check in to see if I was okay, to see that there was no big health issue. But, like opening Pandora's box, all of the demons were about to come out.

November ninth. I remember the day as if it were yesterday. The sun was shining over the Andes mountain range that surrounded the city. The clouds were white and puffy like cotton candy. As I got home from school, I quickly changed into some red pants and a white shirt as I was dragged by my mother into the car. Although the day couldn't have been brighter, I had a dark and muggy feeling inside. We sat in the waiting room for about twenty minutes before the doctor was able to see us, and at first glance, I thought everything would be okay.

Don't worry. They won't change your diet. You aren't sick.

The lady standing in front of me was in her late fifties and had bony hands decorated with extravagant rings and jewelry.

"Come in," she said as she beckoned us forward, opening the door to a spotless office with white walls and a large glass mural with pictures of friendly fish. "Now, let's get down to business. Why are you here?" I wanted to answer that I was asking myself the same thing, but I exercised restraint and told her my parents' concerns. My mother was on the edge of her seat, ready to intervene at any moment if the slightest detail was missing. The doctor's hands raced on the computer keyboard as she typed in all of my information.

Once I ran out of things to say, she ordered me to take my clothes off. I looked at my mom with a surprised expression. I thought we were here to discuss my diet. My mother looked back at me with a stern face that told me I better do as I was told. With trembling legs and unsteady hands, I removed every piece of clothing except my underwear. My red pants and white shirt fell to the floor, wrinkling. I felt completely exposed and vulnerable, a feeling I had not had in a long time.

For many weeks I had enjoyed complete control over my food, and I was feeling great. Finally, after years of being chubby and unathletic, I was on the other side of the equation. Then, the doctor stood up from behind the desk and opened another door. In front of me was the reflection of a pale girl with slumped shoulders and insecure arms that covered her middle section. I couldn't look at myself. I couldn't bear to look at my horrible white, yellowish skin or my soft, mushy belly. Instead, I looked out the window, which was covered by green trees. I observed the leaves and their movement in the wind, the trunk dense and dull.

"What do you see?" the doctor asked, turning her head from the image to face me directly.

"I see myself; it's a mirror," I bluntly responded.

"Do you think you are fat? Thin? Tall? Short?" she asked, squeezing me like a wet paper towel until the last bit of information seeped out of me.

"I think I'm fat. I don't think I am tall or short." At that moment, I wasn't able to formulate sentences. Everything spilled out in monosyllables.

"Do you like what you see?" she asked. I felt as if she were pushing me to the edge of a cliff I hadn't noticed I was walking toward.

"No." There, I said it.

"Okay, then. Come over here and sit on this bed. I am going to take your pressure and listen to your heartbeat.

Still paralyzed with shock by the rush of cold I was feeling, I walked toward the bed, looking back to see my mother with her hands covering her eyes. Still bare and unprotected, I sat on the bed as the doctor attached all sorts of contraptions to my body. She strapped the blood pressure meter to my right arm and clipped on a pulse oximeter to my left index finger. As all of the machines beeped, she grabbed her stethoscope and pressed it against my chest and back.

I closed my eyes and tried to control my breathing, but I was either making things worse or my efforts to seem healthy weren't working. I am not sure why I did this; for all

I knew, I was in perfect condition. It is scary how authority can make you cower, even though you know you've done nothing wrong. Maybe I was frightened by the authoritative figure confirming the reality of what was happening to me.

I can't describe the fear that came over me at that moment. I felt a closing sensation around my chest, even though I knew I was healthy—why wouldn't I be? She shook her head and closed her eyes. Something wasn't right. Taking a deep breath, the doctor looked back at the machines and muttered an obscure sentence that meant things definitely weren't going well.

"Ya po," she finally said. "Put your clothes on." Now, it was she who seemed to articulate in monosyllables.

"I need you to go straight to the cardiology department and get an echocardiogram and ultrasound of your heart. You have lost so much weight that there is not enough fat in your body to use as energy; your body has started eating up muscles. The heart is a muscle, and based on your palpitations, you have been using that muscle as an energy source."

"What does that mean?" my mom blurted out.

"Well, in simple terms, your heart rate is extremely low. About thirty-six beats per minute when it should be sixty to eighty. This means that your heart could stop. Period. Or that you might faint, hit your head, and end up in a worse condition. Hopefully, your situation isn't advanced enough to leave a scar on your heart, but to know for sure, you have to get the tests done. I am booking you an appointment right now. It'll give you time to walk over to the cardiology unit. We need those results today to see what our next steps should be."

My mother and I both nodded and got up quickly from our chairs. Like wild animals released from a cage, we shot out of the office and ran to get the necessary scans. Tears were streaming down my cheeks, curving on my chin, and flowing down my neck. I had no idea what was happening. I had been exercising for the past couple of months and felt nothing out of the ordinary. How could it be that my heart could stop at any moment?

"I'm sorry," I gasped, uttering words whenever my breath allowed. "I know you warned me. I'm sorry." I looked at Mom. I needed to hear her voice.

"You could die," she answered. "My little girl could die."

My mother trampled onto the cardiology floor like a madwoman, waving the paper, which listed the name of the exams I had to take, in the air. In less than fifteen minutes, I was in yet another doctor's office; however, this one had no light and all of the curtains were shut. A big machine with countless buttons and what seemed like a joystick loomed in front of me.

"Take off your clothes," a voice commanded from behind the machine. A short nurse with white plastic shoes assured us that the doctor would be with us soon.

I had the strange feeling of everything moving so quickly that I couldn't fully understand what was happening. The world in my head was slowing down. I heard the buzz of all of the machines in the room, the shuffling of my mother's feet, and a phone ringing in the distance at the main counter. I noticed so many things, yet there was no space in my head to make sense of a situation like this.

When would I have ever thought that I would end up in an emergency room waiting to see if my heart was about to stop? When would I have ever believed I could cause so much pain to my mother? I had never thought about my health or how I had taken my body to such extremes. I didn't think about how much I was hurting myself, possibly sabotaging my future. Would I go to college? How would my father react? What in the world was happening? This was something that happened to others. It was like the plot of a TV drama or a salacious rumor spread on the internet. This wasn't supposed to happen to *me*.

The doctor finally came into the room and told me to lie on the bed. She put a clear cream on the left part of my lower chest and started scanning my heart with a sensor. In a matter of seconds, I saw a black and white picture of my heart beating slowly and rhythmically. The doctor explained that there weren't any scars, which meant the damage wasn't permanent. The thing they were most worried about was the slow palpitations, which meant I was at high risk of fainting and getting dizzy. My mind was whirling with information I had never thought of hearing. My mom simply shook her head and sighed.

"See, Mom? We have to look at the positive side of things. At least it's not permanent."

"Yes," the doctor interjected, "it is not permanent, but you still have to take care of yourself. I am simply doing the scan, but your nutritionist is going to analyze the results. Just to give you a heads up, for the next couple of months, you are probably going to have to see a specialized cardiologist simply to keep track of the progress. Situations like this are very delicate."

My mother gathered the courage to talk and simply asked, "Where can we take the next exam?"

"The next thing you need to do is head over to the room parallel to this and take the echocardiogram. It won't take long."

Both of us nodded, and as I put my clothes on, my mother raced out of the door, desperate for more answers.

HEART ON THE LINE

The next exam simply required some sensors to be placed on specific parts of my chest. It did not take long, but the clack, clack of the printer reporting the condition of my heart made the time pass as slowly as a sea turtle on land.

We went back and forth from one office to the next, consulting with many doctors. Everyone told us that we were lucky we had caught the problem in time, but I didn't feel very lucky.

At last, it was time for the final diagnosis, and from the face of the doctor, you could see that there was no time to waste. She walked us into her office and told us that the exams I had just taken confirmed what she had believed. My heart was beating at an abnormally slow rate, and she recommended ten days off from school. She said that I should not even get up from bed, for the energy that takes could result in darkness. In addition, I was to go see a cardiologist every couple of weeks until my heart was healthy once again.

After explaining in detail everything that needed to change, from my breakfast, snacks, lunch, and dinner, she looked at my face, contorted with tears, and said, "You are going to have to go to a psychologist because your health problems are related to your mental health. You have what is called an eating disorder. What is coming is not going to be easy, but I have a team of great doctors who are going to help you." I would have to see a nutritionist, cardiologist, psychologist, and psychiatrist, all at the same time. I was at a loss for words. In a moment like this, how would you react?

As for me, I simply turned around and cried. I sobbed like I never had before. I looked to my mother every once in a while, hoping for reassurance, but I never found it.

The ride home was quiet, with nothing to be said. Before we left the clinic, I told my mother I couldn't miss ten days of school. I promised her that if I felt anything, I would come straight home. In the end, she agreed, but she would not allow me to participate in physical education.

A million questions clouded my mind: How would my father react? Would he be mad? Why didn't I pay attention to what was happening when I still had control? That day was a day when I experienced many emotions I hadn't felt in a long time. Confusion ripped through my mind, disrupting my thoughts. Guilt was a hurricane that drowned all my peace. I felt like a complete failure. That afternoon, a new leaf bloomed in my mind, and the sky turned a misty gray.

The next day as I walked to school, I felt as if everyone's eyes were on me. Even though the only thing that had changed was that I now knew of my illness, I felt like a completely different person. I nervously walked into class and was greeted by my friends, as always. We had morning class like every other day, and we had our breaks as usual, but something had changed in me. I was cautious with every move I made, not knowing if I would faint, fall, or break a bone. My eyes were those of a paranoid person, protruding out of my skull, scanning for threats. I felt insecure every movement.

Despite this turmoil within me, my first few periods of class passed without any trouble. From what I had observed, nobody suspected a thing. The first break started, and I forced myself to get used to my prescribed food plan. I wanted to throw away all the food my mom packed, to get rid of the calories and never see the snack again. But every time I thought of restricting, I remembered my mother's disappointed face, all the light gone from her eyes. I had to eat for her, for my father, for my brother. I took one painful bite at a time, noticing how my teeth sounded when munching on the granola bar that had 190 calories, noticing how the cool, 80-calorie yogurt felt sliding down my throat.

Abruptly, I felt a horrible pain in my chest, as if someone was stinging me with a needle all around my upper body. I felt like I couldn't breathe. As I inhaled, the invisible needle pierced into my chest; with my exhale, two more needles penetrated the other half. In an act of desperation, I ran to my locker and dialed my mother, trying to explain everything that was happening. Why had I never felt anything like this before? Was my heart about to stop? Even though the school nurse said there didn't seem to be a problem, I found myself in the car heading home thirty minutes after the poison in my chest subsided. The game had just started, and I was losing.

Teachers, parents, and friends often describe a voice in their head that tells them what to do and what not to do. Even at church, the priest encourages you to hear the angel in you instead of the devil. But when it came to my head and the voices I heard, nothing can actually describe the experience of the relentless eating disorder thoughts that plagued my mind.

Every moment of every day, my thoughts revolved around food or what time I was supposed to eat. When I was first diagnosed with an eating disorder, I was sure I didn't hear voices. I wasn't crazy, after all. Yet, as time started passing, I started noticing the unhealthy thoughts:

Throw that ice cream away.

What do you need to drink that yogurt for?

And as the eating disorder consumed me or, let me say, as I let the voice consume me, the thoughts started getting worse:

What would it be like if I didn't exist?

Would anyone miss me?

The voice inside me got so powerful that it forced me to cry every day simply to show people how grave the situation was. I know that the phrase "the voice made me" sounds outlandish, but it's true. If it weren't for those thoughts, I would not have become depressed. If it weren't for those thoughts, I wouldn't have "accidentally" dropped half of the granola bar I brought to eat at school. If it weren't for those thoughts, I wouldn't have simply wet my lips with the yogurt to later throw it away.

About a month went by as every day I "unintentionally" left a bit of food or dropped a bit of my snack, simply letting the eating disorder consume me. I had no energy to fight it off, and after all, my gut said to throw the food away, so why shouldn't I obey? But then again, another voice told me this was wrong. I had heard what the doctor said. Slowly, out of the blue, my anxiety rose every time I got rid of the food. I knew I shouldn't be doing it, and for the first time in my life, I was keeping secrets from my mom.

Ever since I was a little girl, as a family, we had cultivated a dynamic of trust and honesty, an integral part of our family life dynamic, which I had never disrupted, until now. I started feeling a gut-wrenching pain knowing that I was betraying my parents' trust. Now that I had started throwing away food, I was sure they would get mad and be disappointed. I was afraid they wouldn't forgive me, but I couldn't continue feeling the guilt I was feeling. Finally, I decided I was going to open up.

That day after school, I came home and practiced my normal routine. I went upstairs to cry, hoping to get attention.

I wanted my parents to see that I wasn't making any of this up, that the pain swallowing me was all too real. In hindsight, I know that I cried because I was miserable but also because I was seeking compassion and reassurance. Crying, of course, was not the best way to find what I was looking for. So, as I did my homework and then ate, my mind was working as fast as a bullet, trying to find a way to tell my mom what I had been doing without triggering a bomb.

"Mamá," I said, "I have something to tell you." The story came pouring out of my heart. Tears dripped down my face like the crumbs of the granola bar that fell to the floor when I dropped it. When I finished, I looked to my mom. I needed to hear her voice. I needed to know that she forgave me, yet I knew that I wasn't going to get off the hook that easily.

Not a word escaped my mother's lips.

"Are you mad? Sad? What are you feeling?" I pressed.

"I'm in shock. I'm disappointed."

"I'm sorry!" I bellowed. I had triggered a bomb, not in my mom but inside myself.

"I'm sorry. I'm sorry. I'm sorry. I'm sorry." I kept repeating those words as if saying them more often would give them more meaning.

"What can I do so you stop throwing food away?" my mom asked.

"Nothing! I swear I will stop!" I said, not knowing that it wasn't in my hands.

"Let's find a way I can help."

"Maybe I can simply leave the part I normally throw away in my lunchbox so you can see how much I would like to get rid of. When I get home from school, you'll see it, and you can tell me if I should eat it or not."

"Okay," my mom answered, "let's do that."

"Can I have a hug?" I asked, and my mom immediately opened her arms. I pressed my head on her chest and looked at the mirror facing us. I could see three bones sticking out of the back of my neck, something like the spikes of a stegosaurus.

For distraction, my mom and I watched *The Ellen Show* each afternoon, and as Ellen scared Andy, she also scared my thoughts away, at least for a minute. I was going to do my best. I was going to try harder to get better. And I did, but as Christmas drew closer, the ability to fulfill any promise I had made seemed beyond my grasp.

5

CHILE-CARTAGENA: THE MOST WONDERFUL TIME OF THE YEAR

I t was early December, supposedly the jolliest time of the year, but my life was going downhill, spiraling into darkness. Every day I had been eating the same dry chicken and one cup of rice, and my mom decided it was time to change. As I sat down at the dining table, I noticed everything around me: how the light shined on the napkin box, the sizzling of the chicken in the pan, and then the footsteps of the food being brought to the table. In front of me was one cup of lentils and chicken.

I froze. It had been a long time since I had eaten anything different than what was on my "safe" menu. I looked from the plate to my mom again and again. I picked up the spoon and started eating the lentils, but as soon as I finished them, I stood up, walked out of the kitchen, and found a hideout spot that I would use for days to come. Right next to a desk and a wall was a little hole big enough to fit a person. I climbed in and sat there, my back facing the open space and my face staring at the wall.

"Carolina, come here and finish your food!" my mom beckoned, but I didn't answer. "I am going to count to three," she said sternly, as if I were a five-year-old child.

I didn't move. I closed my eyes. Everything went silent. I didn't move and neither did my mom. You could hear a pin drop.

"I am not going to eat that. It's too much," I said, and as soon as I finished speaking, I started bawling.

Saturday and Sunday passed, and I stayed in my hole, my only protection from the outside world. Food was brought, and I would eat it, but not before screaming that I didn't want it.

Monday came and went. The week droned on, and finally, it was Thursday, the first day I was supposed to go to my psychologist. The car ride was the longest trip I had ever taken. Cars zoomed by, each driver living a different life, thinking about different things. Who would have thought that one car held an eleven-year-old girl heading to a counsellor because of her anorexia nervosa?

My mother and I entered a building that looked more like an office than a counseling center. We parked our car and quietly went up the elevator; not a word was spoken. Nerves flowed through my veins and worry made me shiver, my body strongly responding in the minutes, seconds even, it took us to approach the office door. I slowly broke my hand away from my mom's to knock on the door.

Knock. Knock. Knock.

Never had I heard that sound so clearly. Footsteps approached the door, and a small, thin woman let us in. She had wild black hair, and her eyes protruded from their sockets. She wore a long, colorful skirt and a big, black shirt with another loose, long sweater on top. Her hair was in a half bun, and it seemed as if she hadn't slept for days. She said she was pleased to meet me and that I should stay outside in a small reception area while she talked to my mother. I looked around, sinking into the brown and decaying sofa, looking at the paintings on her wall and trying to figure out what they meant. The signature at the bottom said the counsellor's name; she was also an artist.

I stayed for about thirty minutes, scanning the room, reading my book, and trying to hear snippets of the conversation they were having inside her office. Finally, I heard their dreaded footsteps again, and I knew a new battle was about to begin.

"Hi, Carolina! I'm sorry for making you wait. I was talking to your mom about your health details," she said. I simply responded with a forced smile and a blunt nod.

The room was very small, filled with couches, chairs, and pillows. She sat on the biggest, fluffiest chair like a queen on her throne. I sat on the far end of a long, white couch. As I sat, I fidgeted with my hands, plucking the skin on the borders of my nails, digging out the cuticle. The counsellor looked intently at me, but I wasn't able to look back at her.

Time seemed to pass more slowly since the eating disorder ordeal started, and I was suffering. I wondered if something with a greater power, maybe God, wanted to see me in pain. If God is such a generous, kind being, why would he let a person hurt so much? Did I deserve it? What did I ever do?

"So, Carolina, your mom told me her version of the events that have occurred. Now I need you to tell me yours."

"Um," I muttered, "well, I've always wanted to be thin. My family members are really obsessed with being slim and fit, yet I never was. I started eating less and exercising more, and now apparently I have an eating disorder."

"Okay . . . but how do you feel about it? Sad? Frustrated?" She pulled out cards with cartoon faces depicting certain emotions and gave them to me, asking me to explain my feelings with the cards. I looked at her with a weary expression, but I knew I had no choice but to grab the stupid cards and do as she said.

"Well, before, I was a happy girl," I said, slowly pulling out the card with a smiley face. "I would laugh and enjoy everything. My family called me Chinche when I acted like that." The counsellor smiled, expecting me to return the smile, but she was disappointed.

"Can you tell me what Chinche means?" she asked.

"It just something they would call me when I got really excited. I would run around like a puppy and would laugh a lot. Basically, I'd forget everything and just be a little girl."

She looked at me with a face contorted by confusion. I had seen that face on too many people; it didn't bother me anymore. Nothing did.

"Well, Carolina," she started, "I'm glad you don't do that anymore. After all, you are already eleven years old; you can't act like a little child. You are in a very hard moment, and you should be sad all the time. Don't even try to hide it. Imagine me acting like an 'excited puppy.' That would be weird, wouldn't it?"

My eyes opened in surprise. All my life, my parents had told me that I acted too much like a grown up, that I should relax, but if the counsellor said I should be serious and sad, I had to believe it. If I didn't believe her, who could I really trust? I didn't reply to what she said. I simply nodded.

As the session went on, she asked me questions, and I answered. After an endless hour, I was finally allowed to leave. I felt thunder in my veins and lightning in my chest.

You can't act like a child.

You should be sad.

It's going to be okay.

Weeks passed and the drums played the same rhythm. Each day, new leaves grew on the tree that was my eating disorder. Christmas was approaching, and it was time to go back to my one and only home: Cartagena. After all the commotion of the past few months, I couldn't wait for a break. I couldn't wait to see my family because everything was going to be okay. I had to convince myself: everything was okay.

One day, I came home from school in a jittery and anxious mood. I ran to my room and changed into my work out clothes. Before I was banned from exercising, I had forced myself to jog three kilometers three times a week. I would do this rain or shine, and the problem was that I did it because I knew it was one of the best exercises to lose weight. Of course, once they identified my heart issues, I couldn't jog anymore. Nevertheless, I went up to my mom and pleaded for her to let me go out for a jog. I claimed that I needed to run to distract myself and burn off energy, but what I really wanted to do was burn calories. My mom agreed, but only if I limited my run to twenty minutes.

I left the house and set out on the route I used to follow all the time. Abruptly, I felt my legs failing. I tried to think through my movements, one leg in front of another and so on. Every step I ran forward, I felt as if I were falling. I finally decided that I had to go home because it had gotten to the point where I couldn't even walk. I ran into my parents' room bawling. I explained everything to my mom, and she immediately made an appointment with my cardiologist. What had happened was one of three things: either I didn't have enough food inside me to keep me alive and also burn the energy needed to exercise or my heart was failing or it was purely psychological. To this day, I don't know what happened.

When we traveled from Chile to Colombia, I had butterflies fluttering in my stomach. Would my family tell me I was too fat? Would they tell me I was too thin? Are they going to think I'm ugly? Pretty? A thousand worries coursed through my mind, but at last, we got to the Rafael Nuñez airport in Cartagena.

We collected our bags and ran outside to meet our family. Of course, our welcoming committee would not fail us. My aunt, cousin, and grandma were all there. As I embraced my aunt, she looked at me with an examining eye, but she kept her mouth closed. I will always live with the question of what she was going to say, but that is another answer I will never get.

I decided that the best way to cope with my stress and anxiety was to seclude myself, not actually leaving my cousins and family but simply remaining in my room for hours on end reading many, many books. In three weeks, I read eleven books. One day, I was in my mother's room reading, of course, and apparently, my aunt started looking for me. She was yelling, screaming my name, but I was so engrossed in the book that I did not hear her calling me. Suddenly, she walked into the room and started screaming at me.

"Why didn't you answer? I was calling you! I got so worried. Don't you dare do that to me again!" she yelled, tears filling her eyes. It was only years later that my mother told me what had really happened. My aunt was looking for me, didn't find me, and slowly walked toward the balcony. Trembling, she looked down at the ground, five stories beneath us. She thought I had jumped. She was scared. I was scared.

To this day, I do not know if my parents had told my family that I was having suicidal thoughts or if my aunt just sensed there was something wrong.

Endings can't be forced, just as we can't plan for change. That Christmas I was about to learn that we cannot mark our calendars and expect life to be different after a certain day, as many of us do.

It was New Year's Eve, and I was in Cartagena. Every year had been the same. The grown-ups went to a party, and my brother, cousin, and I stayed in my grandmother's apartment. 2016 had been a hectic year, full of happiness and sadness, anger and peace. My world had suddenly turned upside down in an irreversible way. I saw December 31 as a day that would change everything. That day was magical. At midnight, every human being was going to be able to change and follow their New Year's resolution. It was my chance to leave all the trouble behind and begin with a clean slate.

I had a jumpy feeling in my stomach the whole day. I waited attentively all day long. When all the grown-ups left for their annual party, I sat upright in my grandmother's bed and waited, waited, waited. Everyone around me had fallen asleep, but I wasn't about to give in.

After an eternity of waiting, two minutes were left until my life would change. I woke my cousin and brother up and dragged them to the balcony where we would be able to appreciate the fireworks: six, five, four, three, two, one!

There wasn't any wind, but I could feel the salt in the air, intertwining in my hair like a two dancers performing. People were walking along the sidewalk with empty suitcases, thinking that by doing this, the new year would bring them much travel and fortune. Everyone was hoping that the new year would bring them happiness, that their reservoir of joy would grow. I was no exception.

The bay lit up with celebration coming from every corner of the street. Cars honked their horns, and people blew whistles, all in celebration of the new year. Blue, red, gold, and pink, the fireworks were as close as I would ever get to real stars. The people on the bottom floor of the apartment were all dressed up, dancing and singing, and for the next few hours, they would forget all of their worries—until the new year exposed the challenges ahead.

I looked around with a glint in my eye. My brother was looking at the horizon while my cousin was texting all her friends. Everything was exactly the same as it was a minute before. I had made myself believe that my fate would change just because a new year had come. I tried to tell myself that everything was okay, but deep down, I was disappointed, then angry. How could I believe that all the problems I had had during the year would just disappear after the clock struck midnight?

The month went by with fights, screams, and negotiations. Every night when they would serve my cup of rice and chicken, I would eat the chicken and leave small bits, but then I would spread the rice all over the plate as I used to do in kindergarten to make it look as if I had eaten. I asked our helpers to give me less food. I took the chocolate chips out of the granola bars, one by one. Every morning when I had Milo (chocolate milk), I would always leave half of the cup so that they would throw the rest away. It was all a vicious cycle, going round and round, spiraling around me to the point I felt I was suffocating. My mother had all of the stress of the world on her shoulders, with my grandmother's forgetfulness, my disease, and the pressure of our fights.

CHOCOLATE AND OTHER PREDICAMENTS

One afternoon, still enjoying our winter vacation, everybody decided to go down to my aunts' house to eat an afternoon snack.

"Mom," I said, anxiety already building up inside of me, "what do I do?"

"I'll go down. You stay up here and eat your cereal bar. When you are finished, come down, okay?" I nodded, already concocting a method to eat fewer calories.

As soon as my mom disappeared into the elevator, I went into her room and opened the drawer in which she stored all of my snacks. I picked the ninety calorie Quaker cereal bar with the chocolate chips.

Chocolate is bad for you. It makes you fat. Don't eat it.

I unwrapped the cereal bar and looked at the chocolate chips sticking out of it like spines that would cut my throat if I swallowed them. I went into the bathroom and took each chip out, one by one, and wrapped it in a napkin. Technically, I was still eating, and technically my mom never said I couldn't take the chocolate out. I felt a huge satisfaction growing inside of me. Finally, something was in my control.

I had lost every ounce of independence once I had been diagnosed. I couldn't eat by myself, I couldn't choose what to eat, and finally, without consulting anyone, I had won against the calories. I would never let chocolate hurt me, and if the cereal bar was ninety calories before the expulsion of chips, now it would be about fifty calories.

I walked out of the bathroom as if I were leaving a crime scene, not thinking about how I was once again betraying my mother, once again letting my body rot. It didn't occur to me that I simply could not trust myself. I have learned that with having anorexia, one becomes obsessed with control: controlling your emotions, controlling food, controlling hunger, going as far as to ignore it.

After the haunting vacation in Cartagena, we went to Disney as a celebration for our good work during the school year, but I knew that it was only because my parents wanted to see me smile. My twelfth birthday was celebrated by my family, but I didn't care much about it anymore. We went to Cinderella's castle, and for the first time in eight months, I let myself jump and smile when I entered Harry Potter World at Universal Studios. I didn't act like this anymore because, according to the counselor, it was embarrassing and childish. I couldn't be childish. I was twelve years old, after all.

Spinning Teacups, Splash Mountain, and Hogwarts, what more could I ask for? Right? I even had the chance to see Tom Felton, Matthew Lewis, Warwick Davis, and Jason Isaacs, stars of the Harry Potter movies. It was all a dream come true, but if only I could have been myself, my true, pre-eating disorder self. Those two weeks were the happiest I had been in months, but like everything, it eventually came to an end.

For some inexplicable reason, I still couldn't be myself. I was set on the idea that I had to be sad, that I didn't deserve happiness for all the pain I made my family go through. It all came to a point when I no longer knew the true "me," just like I had forgotten what feeling hungry felt like, just like I had forgotten what it felt like to laugh until your stomach hurts. This illness completely consumes you, consuming the person you once were. The things that once brought joy become unimportant events. The monster in my head told me not to eat because it was eating me.

It was one of those horrible days—a day when you can't get up from bed, can't shower, can't brush your teeth, can't open your eyes. I was exhausted from the war raging in my head. I stayed in my room the entire Saturday morning, acting as if I was asleep so I could miss breakfast, but this ruse didn't last long. The nutritionist was not letting me wake up late *precisely* because I would miss breakfast. My mom walked in and lovingly kissed my forehead, but it was no time for love.

"I was asleep!" I scowl.

"Yes," my mom answered, and based on her tone, I knew that she did not have patience to deal with me today. "I know you were asleep, but you have to come and eat breakfast."

"You just want to control my every move. You are happy I am sick. I just proved you right, and the only thing you do is gloat about it!" I yelled, starting a fight.

"Don't speak to me like that," my mom said, her tone rising.

"It's just so unfair. What if I don't want to eat? I don't want to gain weight, and you are feeding me like a pig who's going to take center stage on the Christmas dinner table!"

"Stop this nonsense! You know I love you and am trying to help you!" My mom finally broke, yelling her lungs out.

"I'm sorry for making your life hell. I am sorry for making you want to run away. If it makes you feel better, I can just leave and then you won't have to deal with me!" I screamed, letting my first tears of the day spill down my cheeks and stain my pajamas like transparent blood.

"This is not your fault," my mom replied. "And stop being so unfair with me. If something happens to you, my life will end. I won't be able to take care of your brother, and I will die of a broken heart, so stop!"

"Why do you love me? I am a monster! I have destroyed our lives and created more problems. Everything would be easier if I didn't exist!"

My mom walked out of the room. I had tipped the scale, and she couldn't handle it anymore. After a few seconds, I heard the engine of our car revving, and I watched as my mom left. Rage lifted me up from my bed, and I ran outside, only to find my mom parked at the entrance of our condominium reading a book.

"You left me. Why do I always have to go after you? Why do you run away when I'm at my worst? I am in a dark hole. I am falling, and you are the only thing I am holding on to. I am only alive because of you, and now you run away?"

"I'm sorry," my mom said. "I love you."

"You can't love me. I am a monster." In an instant, the seething waves of my emotions died down.

"I'm just so tired," I cried, "so, *so*, tired. I can't do this anymore. I just can't."

The only thing my mom could do was hold me.

6

CHILE: SHAKING INSIDE OUT

After winter break had ended, my parents sat me down and sternly announced that I was going to go to a psychiatrist. *No. Why, when, who, how?*

Their announcement was an order. I wish I could give more details, but I blocked out that period of my life. I do know that I still sat in my hidey holes. There were two main places where I hid. The one in the dining hall and another on the second floor where I would hide if the dining room wasn't an option. Said hole was between a couch and a table, in the corner of our living room. I would take my books, computer, and phone—sometimes only my thoughts— and I would stay there as long as I could before my parents would drag me out. I still bargained and fought, but I don't remember much more.

Eventually, the day came. I was going to see the doctor. I was hurried out of school, and we quietly drove to the

German Clinic, the place of my nightmares. That hospital had become my second home, an abusive one. Every time I walked through its doors, bad news came shooting toward me: pneumonia, low blood pressure, muscle inflammation, eating disorder, heart failure. We went up the stairs and my hands became fidgety, as if I was holding a bowl of lava that had to be moved from one hand to another, but instead of lava, it was my mother's hand.

As soon as we walked in, I saw a tall man in his early forties with a white coat and hair plastered with gel. As with every doctor I had gone to in the past few weeks (the count was up to five), they all asked about me, what I liked, how I felt. It was a long speech that went on and on, but I had already memorized my answers. I didn't have the energy to adapt my answers based on the day or my mood.

After what seemed like an hour, we finally got to the topic of interest: medicine. I told him that I was not taking any medication and that my dad was not very fond of medicines. After all, I wasn't crazy.

He then went into another long spiel about how coming here didn't mean you were crazy, it meant you needed help. Blah. Blah. Blah. He examined me head to toe and explained the functions of the brain. Blah. Blah. Blah. After about forty-five minutes of pure doctor jargon, he finally told me the medicines I had to take.

"So, for your anxiety, you are going to take two pills every night. For your depression, you are going to take two and a half pills alongside the ones for your anxiety. Oh, and you also told me you are having trouble concentrating in school, so I'll give you a vitamin you have to take every day as well, two tablets."

After he finished listing all of the medicines, my jaw dropped. I looked at my mom. Her face looked surprised, but she tried to contain her thoughts and simply nodded along. Yes, I had to take six and a half pills daily, but after all, we were in the hands of a professional. Everything was going to be okay.

That very night, the pill regimen started. My mother helped me cut all the pills, and life went on. It was my first day of school with medicine in my system. To be honest, I didn't feel a difference because I had never let any of my friends know that I was crumbling, so I simply kept a smiling face and moved on. After having dinner, I was in my little hole in the dining room until I heard my dad come in. I climbed out and greeted him with a hug. What I loved about the hole was that I was squished between the wall and a piece of furniture. I felt secure.

We walked into the kitchen and that's when it all started. I felt my legs shaking violently. Was my heart failing? Was I about to faint? What was happening? I stood near the fridge, holding on to a nearby counter. I started swinging one of my legs back and forth quickly so that my parents wouldn't see that I was shaking.

My dad looked at me with a quizzical face. "Are you okay?" he asked.

"Yeah!" I said, flashing a forced grin.

"Are you sure?"

"Yep! Don't worry about me!"

The next day I followed my daily routine. I woke up, showered, went downstairs to eat breakfast, and squeezed all of the cheese out of the grilled cheese and smeared it on a napkin without anyone noticing. I drank almost all the Milo, leaving the part with the bubbles. I got to school, and by now, we were in the second semester. I shoved all of my things into my locker, grabbing the materials I would need for first period. Once I finished, I ran inside directly to the heaters. Chile can get extremely cold during winter time, but outside, one can observe the Andes Mountains covered with snow, looking like the resting place of angels.

A few minutes later, my advisory and language arts teacher walked in. She was the substitute teacher for this semester because our original teacher was having a baby. Schools always aim for advisory to be a safe place, one where you can joke around and have fun, yet Ms. Ana had been the only teacher who truly helped me feel that way. She always walked into the classroom with a story to tell and a lesson to teach.

That day, we were working on our social justice unit, making PSA posters to advocate for something we were passionate about. I sat down in my chair and grabbed a pencil. I was drawing an ocean littered with plastic to create consciousness about pollution. As I started moving the pencil, my hand started shaking. The lines I was trying to draw appeared on the paper like excited worms moving everywhere. I took a step back and breathed. What the heck was happening? I tried once again, yet the same result was in front of me. Not knowing what to do, I resorted to telling Ms. Ana, one of the few people I actually trusted.

"I can't stop shaking," I said, faking a smile so it wouldn't seem so serious. My mother had previously talked to my teachers about what was happening, so Ms. Ana was concerned.

"Have you eaten?" she asked, and I had, if half a cereal bar counts. After realizing there was nothing anyone could do to help me, I shrugged off other suggestions and continued my work.

Then came social studies, a very challenging class that stressed everyone out but was balanced by a great teacher, a person who had been supporting me every step of the way. As I walked in, Ms. Massey told us to sit down and work on writing notes on the South African Apartheid article in front of us.

"You can either write notes on the computer or on paper, but if you want to use the computer, you'll have to wait. For some reason, we are having tech issues again." Everyone smiled and grabbed a paper. As I picked up my pencil and started writing, my hand simply could not move correctly. At that point, my whole body was shaking, and I could barely move my head. Nobody noticed except Ms. Massey. I could feel her gaze on the back of my neck, but she didn't say anything. Now, I knew had to wait for the computer because writing was obviously not an option. The minutes went by as slowly as a slug on the road, and finally, the bell rang. It was time for science.

Before starting sixth grade, I had a middle school buddy who helped me get to know the classes and explained how everything worked: "The order of blocks is going to change every week, but the one thing you should know is that you should *always* run to the cafeteria. The lines can get very long . . . There are two sides, and you definitely don't want to get the white side. Mr. Booth is the science teacher, and you won't want to get him in a bad mood. You know? Once, a boy left his locker open, and Mr. Booth took everything out and stashed it in his classroom . . . Oh, and are you Canadian? If you are Canadian, you won't want to be in his class. He always picks on two people per class, and they are normally Canadian."

The whole tour went on like this. I listened to all of her complaints and strange stories until she got bored and, as many buddies do, left me alone. Yet one thing was clear: I didn't want to be in Mr. Booth's class.

Flash forward to the day after I started taking the pills. I ran out of social studies and into my science class.

"Hey, Mr. Booth," I said, hoping someone in class would get him off task so that he could tell us stories about the Peace Corps and tell us that if you are talking about a group of pugs you should call it a grumble. Thankfully, that day, one of my friends (a Canadian, of course) told us that we had to someway bring up the movie-book controversy. He said that his brother, who had Mr. Booth last year, promised that topic would keep the teacher off track all class long. (He also told us that if Mr. Booth asked us any questions we didn't know the answer to, we should simply say "density.") Somehow, we managed to start talking about movies that are better than books. I, of course, said that books were always better than movies. Mr. Booth looked at me with a face we all knew too well. He was about to talk about *The Princess Bride*.

"*The Princess Bride* is a book and a movie, and the movie is much better!" He rapidly looked up a clip from the movie, one he had already shown us two other times. This was the scene when they were accusing a woman of being a witch. Mr. Booth had used that scene to teach us about both the scientific method and density, and now he was using it to prove some movies are better than the book they are based on.

I exaggeratedly squinted at the screen and the pixelated people moving on the projection screen. Mr. Booth sat on his chair, leaning back with a wide grin. His face was saying, "I told you so!"

"Well," I said, "we wouldn't know if the movie is better than the book because you can barely see the people on the screen! When was this made? 1980?" Mr. Booth looked back in shock. The debate had begun.

He stood up and said, "It was actually made in 1987, but don't worry, I understand what you are saying. You are simply calling me old and outdated, but that's okay." Everyone laughed as Mr. Booth took a seat in front of me.

My cheeks blossomed red, and I immediately tried to explain. "No! That's not what I am saying!"

He just shook his head and looked at me with dismay. He had always had a very good poker face. Suddenly he started blurting out movies: "*Wizard of Oz!*"

"I read the book, and it is much better than that eternal movie," I said

"*Cinderella, Alice in Wonderland, The Little Mermaid,*" he said

"Those books are just plain gory. We are not talking about the kids' version, right?" Everyone laughed, and for a few seconds, I felt good, close to happy: Mr. Booth making his sarcastic comments, my classmates answering, all of it a perfect fit.

The day continued, and I went to math. It was a class I didn't much care for, yet I always felt safe there, knowing my teacher would help me every step of the way.

That very same day during lunch, my friends and I had to go back to Mr. Booth's classroom to work on a special yearbook (that never ended up working). As we entered the room, Mr. Booth sat at a desk with a tray of brownies. From what I had heard, he was an amazing baker. His monster cookies were famous, and my mother couldn't stop begging him for his carrot cake recipe. But how would I know about his baking skills? I never tried anything.

My best friend was already sitting at another desk, gulping down her brownie. I walked toward the tray full of brownies. Everybody in the room was calm, thinking about different things, yet I was about to make the hardest decision of my life. Would I eat the brownie? It had way too many calories, and I was already eating enough things. Nevertheless, I scooped up a brownie and wrapped it in a napkin. Mr. Booth smiled at me, and I went and sat down.

Katrina smiled at me, and I showed her the wrapped brownie. Her gaze motioned to her lunch box, and I placed it inside. Of course I wasn't going to eat the brownie. When those situations arose, I didn't want to be the girl who didn't eat the sweets, but I also was the girl who didn't eat the sweets. Thus, I always gave them to my friends.

The bell rang, and the hallways got crowded with everyone hurrying to get their things and go home. I met my mom outside of school, and she immediately took me to the psychologist. *Of course*, I thought, *it's Thursday*.

We made our way down the far-too-familiar road. I did not utter a word the whole ride. My vision was blurry, my hands were shaking, and I couldn't move my head. Every few minutes, my mom would look back at me through the rearview mirror with a furrowed brow. I knew she wanted to ask what was wrong, but she knew I wouldn't want to answer.

The psychologist was late, and we had to sit on the floor in the hallway, waiting for her to open the door and let us in. Everything seemed to move slowly. One moment, she was walking toward us, and the next, I was already sitting on the couch, listening to her ramble on about being mature and not letting your feelings consume you. I couldn't take it anymore, so I interrupted her and told my mom to come into the room.

"I'm sorry to interrupt your speech, but there is something more important I need to talk about," I said. I started explaining all the events of the day, showing her how I wasn't able to write or even shake my head. I felt like a robot, slowly using up its battery. The counsellor only nodded and smiled while my mom's mouth was wide open in shock.

"Oh," she said, "I see."

"Well, then, what should I do about it?" I asked with a stronger tone than what I had intended.

"See, I'm a counselor," she answered. "I don't know what's wrong with you. You should see your psychiatrist."

The session continued with the same monotony as always. Once it had finished, I stormed out of the counselling room, not wanting to be looked at, touched, or spoken to. I stomped the floor, and the heavy steps vibrated through my whole body. I asked my mom to give me the car keys and ran to climb in the back seat. Before my mom could get in, I started screaming my lungs out.

"Why?" I yelled out loud, not knowing who I was talking to. "Why me? What have I done to deserve this? I just want this to end! I can't take it anymore!" Tears were streaming down my face like whitewater rapids, and the worst part was, I meant everything I said.

My mother came running to the car and simply started driving, hearing me scream as I had never done before, only muttering, "I know, I know."

Once we arrived at home, I saw my dad's car was pulling into the driveway while we were still at the gate of the condominium.

"Stay back here," I pleaded with what was left of my voice. "Dad won't understand why I'm crying."

My mom looked back with genuine worry on her face. "I know you have had a rough time with dad, but you can't keep pushing him away. You may think he won't understand, but he loves you more than anything, and that is what you need at the moment."

We finally walked into the house, and my dad was waiting for us at the bottom of the stairs. "Why did you stay back?" he asked, and immediately tears started streaming down my face.

"I'm so tired, Papi, so, so tired," I said, shaking once again.

"It's okay," he said. "Everything is going to be okay."

I had not realized how much I missed his strong hand stroking my head. Ever since the incident with my caretaker, we had started drifting away. In other words, I started keeping him away. For the first time in a while, I felt safe. I was under the caring wings of my father.

When I was little, I was always worried that a monster would break into the house or, worse, break into my dreams, but my dad was always there, saying he would protect me. Now that the monster was already in my head, he was keeping his promise. His hugs were strong and warm, and his shoulder the perfect fit for my head to lean on. That was the only thing I needed.

After discussing what had happened during the day, we tried to make an emergency appointment with my psychiatrist. For about a week, my mother emailed the clinic, emailed the doctor personally, and called everyone she could, but nobody answered. However, after a week of rage pilling up inside of us all, we were able to book an appointment.

We waited in the familiar reception area and finally heard my name called. As we walked down the hall, we could see my doctor outside of his door, waiting with a huge smile on his face.

"I'm going to kill you," my mom said under her breath, with a big smile on her face, but I knew that she wasn't joking.

"I am so sorry about the delay," he said. "Please, come in."

For the fourth time that week, I explained everything that had happened, reciting every occurrence and alien sensation. His smile never faded, but you could see the worry and regret in his eyes.

"Okay, then," he said, "please stand over here and stick your arm out in front of you." I forced my arm to extend, feeling every single muscle work, something I am not sure you should feel. He started bending my arm as if it were a door. My arm trembled, up and down, up and down. Next, he told me to walk in a straight line. I once again struggled to put one foot in front of the other, but I managed to get across the room without stumbling. For the next fifteen minutes, he moved my head from side to side and made me stand on my tiptoes.

"Well," he finally said. "The good news is this is just an allergic reaction to the medicine. Thankfully there is no neurological damage. One more day with this medicine, and we might have had something worse to deal with." I sighed with relief, not processing the severity of what he had said.

"Your mother knows who I am," my mother said, her voice trembling, making everything shake around her like an earthquake. "She knows that there is a Colombian woman with an anorexic twelve-year-old who has been calling you a son-of-a-bitch ever since this started." And with that last statement, my mom grabbed my arm and pulled me out of the room.

I didn't know what had happened. I wasn't paying attention; I was just breathing. Why is this happening to me? What did I do wrong? Little did we know that he was giving me a highly dangerous drug not recommended for people under eighteen. The doctors we trusted my life to ended up endangering it.

7

CHILE: WITCHES AND BACKPACKS

For the first time, my mom was in a deep state of desperation. She was fidgety, and when I got home from school, her eyes were always puffy because of unspoken tears.

One day, I came home and found my mom on her phone, listening to an audio recording as tears dripped down her face.

"What are you doing?" I asked with genuine concern.

"Nothing," she said as if there was something she needed to hide.

"Mom, I have enough problems without being worried about you. Please tell me what's wrong."

She sighed, nodded, and said, "A few weeks ago, I was having lunch with a friend, and our conversation drifted to spirit mediums."

"Wait, what mediums?"

"Spirit mediums, people who are the link between the creators and mortals."

"But we are Catholic!" I exclaim. "You have never believed in that; we have never believed in that."

"That's beside the point," my mom said. "I contacted her, and she supposedly starting to fix things between us and the universe."

"At least tell me what she said," I replied, rolling my eyes but feeling curiosity burn up inside me.

"She said that in a past life I might have been raped or maybe I died of hunger, and that is why I am so obsessed with you eating."

"Mom, what do you mean you were raped?"

"The medium said in a past life I was raped and that it somehow affected me in this life, but I forgot what she said about it exactly."

"Don't you think you are obsessed with me eating because I have an *eating disorder*, and not because you died of hunger in another life you *don't even remember*?"

"Gorda," she said, tears ready to escape her eyes, "I'm desperate. And I do feel the difference, don't you? Maybe she is talking to the spirits. She better be because these sessions are expensive. I have asked her to read into your past and your father's past, and she told me she is communicating with the spirits in order for our energy to change."

Was something really changing? Was this actually true? Was my mom delusional?

"I don't like this, Mom. Since when have you started believing in magic-hocus-pocus things?"

"I just want you to get better, and if it means having to summon all of the non-existent spirits in the world, I will do so." Chills started creeping up my back, onto my shoulders, and down my torso again, just like in *The Sixth Sense*.

For the following weeks, I convinced myself that I was feeling better, that the spirits were actually helping me, but as time passed, things continued with their normal monotony. My standard medical treatment continued, even though my mom was also getting into this hocus pocus thing.

My mom's actions demonstrate the measures people will go to when they are desperate. Nevertheless, some measures simply don't work, and one just has to keep looking.

INTRUSIVE THOUGHTS

Once again, nothing changed. By that point in time, I had figured out that we were moving to Singapore. At first, my ignorance was so great that I didn't even know where Singapore was on a map. I heard phone calls and conversations about whether or not moving was the right choice. I didn't want to hear or think about it. But I knew what I had to do; I tried to convince my parents that I was going to be okay and that they shouldn't waste this opportunity simply because I was sick. I would feel guilty if I messed this up for my father.

And, deep down, I had the enticing thought that if we moved, there would be new food and maybe I could convince my parents to buy me lower calorie food. When these thoughts came to my mind, I felt as if I were possessed. Ever since I was a little girl, I had always focused on cause and effect. I had always been very mindful of how a situation may turn out if I made a certain decision, yet when the voices worked their evil magic, all logic escaped my body. I was in a trance that no one could take me out of. I simply wasn't there.

As the move drew closer and closer, I sensed the stress building up and creating walls that didn't let us communicate.

Part of the process of admission to my new school in Singapore was to write an application essay that, in simple terms, proved you were good enough to enter. It was a sunny afternoon, and I was walking from class to the car to go home. I walked on the very edge of the sidewalk where the little leaves of grass touched the cement. Abruptly, the strangest thought came to my head: *If you step on that green leaf two steps in front of you, you are not fat. But if you don't, you are.*

Later, I learned these are "intrusive thoughts" and that most people have them. I had always been afraid of telling people that I thought like this because it sounds completely bonkers, but those thoughts were the ones bringing me down. Obviously, before having that thought, I was pondering what would be for dinner and remembering to squeeze the cheese out of the sandwich I would have for breakfast the next morning. I walked steadily forwards, controlling my body as much as I could. I had to touch that leaf. If I didn't, I would be fat and would finally have to give in to the eating disorder. One foot in front of the other, and finally, I stepped on the leaf.

Okay. It's okay. Right? Now I know I'm not fat, right?

I looked at my wrists, my watch dangling alongside my other bracelets. I touched the point of my index finger and thumb together and circled them around my wrist. They could make a perfect circle, but I felt my finger straining a little bit. I knew I had gained weight. Maybe, since my pinkie finger creates a wider circle, I could prove that I was not fat by using pinky and thumb. Thus, I repeated the same process and cuffed my wrist once again. Okay. My wrist fits. It's okay.

I got into the car and gave my mom a hug. Once I felt her soft, warm hands on my shoulder, I started bawling.

"Why is this happening to me? I can't control myself! I didn't want this! I am so sorry!" I cried.

"We are not moving," said my mom,

"Yes, we are! I need to leave this place!"

"But, you have friends and doctors here!"

"Does that make a difference? Look at me! I am a mess! I need help, and I can't find it. I feel so alone. I just want to die!"

My mother looked at me, her face wide in shock. I knew that every time I said I couldn't take the sickness any longer, it meant I was having morbid thoughts, though I had never clearly stated that I was thinking about death. Now, I had confirmed both my fears and those of my family.

We drove home in complete silence, and as soon as I opened the front door, I went to the backyard. I lay face down on the concrete floor of our courtyard, even though I was surrounded by furniture. I took out my notebook and started writing down the application essay for my new school, but I wasn't focusing on the words. I was focusing on how my rib cage felt touching the cold floor, how my pelvis grazed the concrete. My diaphragm contracted and expanded, yet my ribs were still able to touch the floor.

I stopped writing. Temptation had won. Now I was trying to see how many bones could touch the floor. The more they did, the thinner it proved I was. Ribs, pelvis, collarbone, shoulder bone. Okay. It's okay.

However, temptation can end up in addiction. I left all of my school supplies outside and stormed into the house, up the stairs, and into my room. I lay down facing up and tucked my toes in an opening under my bed. I used my abdomen to push me up: one crunch, two crunches, three, four, five . . . twenty. Now it was time for push-ups: one push up, two push-ups, three, four, five . . . twenty. Now wall squats: two minutes. Now the plank: two minutes.

Then, I Googled five-minute workouts that burned the most calories. I played the video and followed along, even though I had no idea what calories even were. I just knew they made you fat and that you didn't want them in your body. Even though I was not supposed to be moving because my heartbeat was at thirty-six beats per minute, I felt great—a little dizzy and out of breath, but great.

Maybe now I had burned the calories I had eaten during afternoon snack. If I was lucky, maybe I'd burned my morning snack as well. After all, the only thing the eating disorder wanted to eat was me and my peace of mind.

My anxiety heightened exponentially. Every time any doubtful thought entered my mind, I grew fidgety. My fingers were raw flesh because every time my anxiety took over, I would pick off the skin on the border of my nails, so the pain in my fingers was constant. My lips were always dry and chapped, and my boney toes were always scraping against my socks. It's a miracle I never plowed a hole through my socks. Anxiety may be a mental illness, but if you let it go too far, it can cause physical symptoms.

Every two years, my whole extended family goes on a trip together. Typically, we go on a cruise through different parts of Europe, but this year was different. Because I had already been sick for a little less than a year and we were about to move to Singapore, my anxiety was reaching record heights. So, my parents decided it was better to stay behind this time. This caused my mother great stress because, on top of dealing with my eating disorder, my mom also wanted to be with her mother, who was suffering from dementia, as much as she could. So, my grandma got on an airplane and came to Chile.

At first everyone was happy, finally seeing our grandmother. She represented safety and normality, something I didn't have in my life. I assumed that life would be just like it was before this hurricane of problems came toward us because my grandma was here and she always made everything seem lighter. Nevertheless, as the week went by, reality sank in as I perceived her deterioration.

We would be in the middle of playing cards with her when she would forget what kind of game we were playing, and all of this hit my mother in a very vulnerable spot. We all tried to be there for her, but as always, it is difficult to act when you don't understand. However, my grandma was lively and happy. All she wanted to do was buy us gifts and make us laugh. Yet, I was in a part of my sickness where my self-esteem was so low that I never accepted anything from anyone.

After all, I didn't deserve any gifts. Why would I? I destroyed my parents' lives by having this eating disorder and pushing my mom into her depression. I would fight and scream whenever my mom came home with a new shirt or a set of pencils. I had hurt them enough; they shouldn't be spending their money on me. I was a monster. Why did they even want me here? Were they planning on abandoning me?

One day, after my mother saw the terrible state my backpack was in, she told my grandmother that they should buy me a new one. Of course, in a normal situation, this would seem like the rational thing to do. But, remember, this wasn't a normal situation.

When I got home, I saw a huge bag with a beautiful new backpack. My body burned. It was as if I could feel the steam leave my ears like in cartoons.

"Mom!" I yelled, and it was as if she teleported into my room because she was standing in front of me in less than twenty seconds.

"Well," she said, a glimmer of hope in her eyes, "do you like it?"

"I didn't tell you to buy me a backpack! I don't want it!" I screamed.

She looked utterly taken aback. "What do you mean? It's a present from your grandmother."

"I don't want it!"

"Why?" she said, raising her voice to match mine, which I couldn't regulate.

"I don't know! I just don't want it!"

"Tell me the truth! Why are you acting like this? It's just a backpack!"

"I don't deserve it, and you know it! Why do you even bother spending money on me? I know you want to abandon me. But you are a good person, and that would affect your conscience, so I will just leave. Then everyone can live in peace. You won't have to cover my expenses, and you won't have to suffer through my problems anymore!"

At that moment, I broke down in tears. My grandmother never found out about my breakdown, how such a small trinket had made me lose all remaining composure.

STARTING OVER

In addition to this huge tree called anorexia blooming in my mind and taking over, we still had the move to consider. After all, Singapore is 18,695 kilometers away from Cartagena, roughly the equivalent of thirty hours on a plane. We were about to embark on a voyage at the very moment our ship was sinking. My parents heavily debated whether going to Singapore was the most prudent decision. I had doctors in Chile, and for what we knew at the moment, they were the only certainty we had.

Before moving to Chile, I was ignored and excluded by my classmates in Colombia. Hence, when we moved, I saw it as an opportunity to start from scratch and present myself as a confident, strong girl. Maybe the same thing could happen with Singapore. Maybe all this turmoil in my head would disappear, or perhaps I would at least learn to manage it better. I don't know what reasoning I used to support this way of thinking, but I thought maybe, just maybe, since the food over there was so different, I could eat less.

8

SINGAPORE: BOXING AND UNBOXING

The move was in full swing. All of the boxes had been packed and sent off to Singapore, and the only thing left to do was say goodbye. For that afternoon, my life was normal. I hung out with my friends. We laughed, made slime, and gossiped, just like any other teenagers would do. Nevertheless, all good things come to an end, and before I knew it, I was on a plane for twenty-seven hours headed to a part of the world unknown to me.

Honestly, I have no recollection of the first few weeks in Singapore, partially because of the jet lag and partially because the time zones were completely different. (Singapore is thirteen hours ahead of Chile.) This means my pill-taking schedules were also off. For all we knew, I might have been taking two doses a day before my body finally adjusted to

Singaporean time. One day, my brother woke up at ten at night thinking it was already morning; in summary, it was a long night for him.

All of these changes created a mountain of anxiety, which came in the form of negotiations and fights with my parents, nightly crying sessions, and an overall a terrible mood. I would cry and scream and pout, not knowing why. Afterwards, I would feel guilty for crying, screaming, and pouting, so I would become anxious and cry and scream and pout all over again. It was a cycle that seemed unbreakable at the time. Nevertheless, my mother had something else on her mind; she wasn't going to let jet lag come in between her and my eating schedule.

One day, I had just woken up (at six at night), and my mother was making dinner. Of course, since I had to fight to get over my fear of food, she was making chicken nuggets. Let's just say that the mitten she was using to get the nuggets out of the oven was not the greatest quality. She reached in the oven and grabbed the scorching hot glass pan. She didn't scream or yell; she held on to the pan because she couldn't ruin my dinner. It did not matter if she lost her hand, at least I would have something to eat. Stubbornly, she kept on holding to the pan until I came running to help her. I snatched the pan and started serving the food, knowing that the only way I could help at that moment was to eat everything on my plate.

Meanwhile, my mother was still in the kitchen, not uttering a word but wearing tears of pain on her face. We called the emergency service, and they came to help her. Later on, she would tell me that she had never felt any physical pain compared to that, but she knew I had to eat. For the following weeks, my mother couldn't use her hand. She had huge white blisters that would randomly ooze pus and then fill up again. All because of me. If it hadn't been for my eating disorder, my mom would have let go of the tray and her burns wouldn't have been so grave. *Why can't I do anything right?* I wondered.

We moved to Singapore in May, but my mother had been looking for doctors since January. She emailed various hospitals, explaining my situation. Nevertheless, they kept referring her to other doctors until she finally got an appointment with both a psychologist and a psychiatrist. The psychiatrist was a leading figure in the eating disorder realm, but a few days after making the appointment, she had to cancel because I was under thirteen; this was disappointing. Even so, we kept the appointment with the psychologist, but the sessions would not start until school commenced.

I had been attending my new school for about a month, and although I had not been able to make friends, I did my best to keep my head held high and my smile shining brightly. Singapore baffled me in every sense of the word. The enormous skyscrapers, decorated with cutting-edge architecture, touched the clouds. Fancy cars rolled down the streets, and every few blocks, one would see people casually lining up to enter a big name-brand store.

By this time, I had been struggling with the eating disorder for about a year and felt I was attached to a heavy chain that wouldn't let me move forward. Getting up in the morning was a challenge. I dragged through the day, hiding as much of my body as possible behind baggy clothes.

Many hold a big misconception about the main issue with eating disorders. They are not simply about eating too much or too little; for me, that was actually the easiest part to cope with. The extreme anxiety and depression, which pull you down like an anchor, are the most distressing elements. I lived in a chronic stage of sadness, but my life droned on.

Moving from country to country didn't make things any easier. It didn't shield me from the tortuous remarks of my classmates. When I moved to Asia, kids took advantage of my weakness and found every flaw that I possessed. My name was contorted until it was unrecognizable, and even though I tried to ignore them, to stand up for myself, it was all useless.

My days became measured in numbers. At six each morning, I'd eat breakfast (four hundred to five hundred calories); then four hours later, I had to eat a snack (about two hundred calories); and then in two more hours, I ate lunch (four hundred to five hundred calories). Mom promised that lunch wasn't more food than normal. "Don't worry," she told me. "You won't get fat."

But what if she made a mistake? Maybe you should leave a little food.

No. You are not going to do that.

You'll see, you will gain weight and become the chubby laughingstock of everyone in the school.

But my parents promised me they would never let that happen.

Oh, come on. How can you be so gullible?

Day in and day out, an omnipotent voice consumed my thoughts. The pills I was taking were supposed to calm the voice and help me think properly. After all, I took one anxiety pill and two other concentration vitamins, but here comes another misconception: pills don't cure anything. This medicine isn't like an Advil you take to make the headache disappear. These pills are simply to give you strength and energy to fight all of the demons around you.

My doctors told me to try and stop the eating disorder from consuming my life. They told me to picture it like a chair in a big room: don't pay attention to the chair; just acknowledge its presence and move on. This seems like an easy task, but when you have a monster inside of you that is consuming every bit of your sanity, you are lifting the weight of the world. I felt like a warrior losing a battle. I could see my mental enemies charge forward with menacing spears and bows, but I couldn't fight them effectively.

My head was so lost and fogged that I started calling the voice by a name. At the time, Harry Potter was my obsession. I lived and breathed the wizarding world, hoping against all odds to be sucked into it as I read. In Quidditch, there is a big, heavy ball called a Bludger whose goal is to knock people off of their flying brooms and leave them injured and defenseless. That was exactly what was living in my head. I tried to knock it away. I tried to be the bigger person and fight back, but when you are fighting against a Bludger you created, things get much more difficult. The game seemed lost.

Just like Eddie Brock in the movie *Venom*, I sensed the voices in my head driving me insane. I tried to justify them, saying it wasn't really me. *I* didn't really want to throw food away, but *the Bludger forced me to do it.* The voices became so loud and persistent that the only way I could drown them out was by finding a bigger distraction.

During a remarkably terrible day, I came home from school feeling my emotions pulling me down. As I entered the house, I threw my backpack on the ground and stormed to my room. Sliding down against a wall, I started crying and crying and crying. I couldn't stop.

You are so fat.

Why are you eating so much?

Your life is a mess.

You are a mess.

Suddenly, I started banging my head against that wall. "Stop!" I yelled. "Stop!" My cries became louder and louder. The voices wouldn't stop. It was as if the only way to stop hearing those incessant voices was to create a more painful sensation that I could focus on instead. *Bang. Bang. Bang.* Tears dripped down my face and pain seared through my skull.

It sounds crazy, but the voices make you think terrible things. I dreaded the weekends, knowing my family would be staring at me every time I ate. Before the eating disorder, I would wake up at ten or eleven each morning. (Toward the beginning of my sickness, I would do this simply not to eat breakfast.) When I was eventually forced to follow my diet more strictly, I would wake up at six or seven in the morning reminding myself that I had to eat breakfast. If I didn't, my body would think I was starving, and it would start saving the fat from the food, making me fat again. There was no way out, and my anxiety wouldn't let me sleep.

I had many clothes in my wardrobe: shirts, shorts, pants, and skirts. But I wouldn't wear most of them because I had certain dress code rules. The shirts had to have sleeves, and I could only wear pants. That is how I started wearing a red shirt and jeans every weekend. I wouldn't wear anything else. I lived in those skinny jeans that looked too baggy on me because they didn't stick to my body. I wore a huge, red t-shirt to hide my belly. Thank God I had two of those shirts and two of those pants; for Saturday and Sunday, my comfort was assured.

Art had become my favorite class. The teacher was the only instructor at my new school who seemed to like me, and I had the liberty of creating whatever I pleased. As I carefully drew the outline of a dove on my canvas, a boy in the class stood up and joined the conversation that the "cool" kids were having.

"OMG, guys," he said, "in English class, all we do in book clubs is talk about how much we hate Carolina."

My heart skipped a beat. I wasn't able to process the pain I was feeling inside my chest. It wasn't as if anyone was dying. Why did I feel such surprise and sadness?

See? I told you!

But I have only been here for two months. I haven't said anything! I eat lunch alone and only speak to participate in class. Why would they hate me so much?

Maybe it's just because you deserve it.

Do you think so?

Of course! Why else would they take the time to bellow it in front of the class? On top of hating you, they want you to know it.

Luckily, the bell rang, and we were dismissed from class. I headed toward my next block, Chinese.

"Wǒ kěyǐ shàng cèsuǒ ma?" May I go to the bathroom?

"Kěyǐ." You can.

I ran to the nearest bathroom and locked myself in one of the stalls. I tried to control my breathing. I knew I was too strong to let petty comments from seventh graders affect me, but I was too deprived of energy to fight against the storm of sadness. Tears flowed down my cheeks, creating a river full of the memories of all the things that had hurt me. Words and insults flowed into my head, punching and kicking at my consciousness.

You are so stupid. Why can't you be stronger? Nobody likes you. Your parents should abandon you. You are causing so much suffering in everybody's life. You shouldn't even exist.

Stop it, please. I can't take it.

What? Can't you take the truth? Accept the mess you are.

I can't.

Do it.

It's not true.

Stop fighting. You know it is.

Okay.

The will to move on was sucked out of me. The sun I had tried so hard to see was being blocked by thunderous clouds. The open wounds that had never healed burned and itched, causing my strength to fade even more. What I wanted to do was clear and simple: I wanted to stay inside the bathroom stall and stop trying to be strong. I wanted to rest. Sometimes, it just seemed easier to let the eating disorder take control. If it did, I didn't have to fight.

However, the image-conscious and determined voice inside my head forced me out of the bathroom stall. I leaned close to the mirror and wiped the poisonous tears. I patted down my disheveled eyebrows and tied up my hair into a neat ponytail. Even in moments like this, when I could feel exhaustion coming out through my pores, I stood on my side and examined my belly.

It's too big. Don't tuck your shirt in.

Okay.

I walked out of the refuge I had created for myself and acted as if nothing had happened. Predators always attack the weak prey first.

9

HONG KONG: LOOPHOLES AND CONCESSIONS

fter a few months of living in Singapore, we finally took our first trip to explore Asia and started with Hong Kong. It was an exciting experience. Before leaving the house, we packed a bag full of snacks in case I didn't like the food. We feared that if I lost any more weight, my heart could stop working again.

We arrived in Hong Kong and drove to our hotel, observing compact buildings in clusters throughout the whole city. Never had I seen so many people together in one place. It was a photographer's paradise. After exploring the city, we went on a tour on the outskirts of the town. We went to a beautiful temple at the base of the Tian Tan Buddha, definitely one of the most impressive things I had ever seen in my life. It was surprising to know that so long ago, with few tools or advanced knowledge, people were able to build such an imposing statue.

We enjoyed the beautiful monastery, learning about the rich traditions and rites practiced in the area. Since it was already late afternoon, we—well, I—had to eat lunch. The tour included a meal at a vegetarian restaurant with traditional cuisine.

I saw this as a chance to not eat. After all, before the eating disorder, I was a picky eater. So, why did that have to change now? They brought plates of spring rolls and other unrecognizable stews. I was forced eat the spring rolls and a cup of rice. Holding back my tears as I felt the greasy layer of deep-fried spring roll was one of the hardest things I had ever done.

Since my brother was also refusing to eat, we left the restaurant. I assumed that we would all simply eat less that day. However, when my mom gets an idea, she will do anything in her power to achieve the goal, and at that moment, her goal was to get me something to eat. We walked through a small market, and my mother's wish came true. A food court plaza appeared with a Subway and a pizza place.

Anxiety built up inside of me, and I knew I was going to have to eat the pizza, that pile of carbs and grease and calories. As fast as lightning, my mother ordered the pizzas, and before I knew it, I was sitting next to my mom, her eyes expectantly drifting from the pizza to my eyes.

"Eat it," she said,

"But I already ate the spring rolls and the rice."

"That was not enough, and you know it."

We kept arguing back and forth until my mom finally said that I would be eating less anyway. A pizza and a few spring rolls was not a good lunch, and it was less than I would be eating if we weren't on vacation. That was what pushed me to eat the pizza. It wasn't my health or my sanity that made me give in. It was the thought of eating fewer calories than normal that made me accept her point.

I wore a long face the whole ride back to Hong Kong; my spiraling thoughts threatened to choke me. As the long road trip ended, we arrived at a gift shop that we had to pass through to get to our van, which would later take us to the hotel. I walked ahead of the group, claiming I needed to go to the bathroom, and when I got out, I saw no one. I walked around, trying to look for my parents, and when I finally saw them, I convinced myself it wasn't them. I convinced myself that they had abandoned me. I ran out of the store like a maniac and started rummaging through my backpack for my phone.

They left without me.

I had it coming.

I knew they would abandon me.

Fear shook every fiber of my body, and I let out tears of anguish. A few seconds later, my parents strolled out of the gift shop.

"Why did you leave me? I thought you had abandoned me!" I said, knowing that I had seen them in the gift shop but preferring to think that they had left me behind. After all, I didn't deserve them, and they didn't deserve this. Like the victims of the Salem witch trials, I convinced myself that something was happening when everything was normal.

"We would never leave you!" my dad exclaimed, scooping me into his arms. "Why would we leave you? You are our everything." That wasn't the only time I convinced myself my parents were abandoning me. It also happened in grocery stores, IKEA, and shopping malls. Everywhere we went was a new opportunity for my parents to relieve themselves of the burden of dealing with me.

Every day had become a routine. After school, I would eat my snack, and a few hours later, I would barge into the kitchen to make rice. Rice is a big part of my family's daily life. We eat rice for lunch and dinner, and we even have a special recipe. You first cut long spaghetti into little pieces and then fry it in oil. Then, add condiments, and finally the rice. However, the day I realized that you had to fry the little spaghetti pieces, I made it my personal goal to get rid of that unhealthy junk. Slowly but surely, I started taking away the oil from the recipe. If my mother noticed, she never said anything, but eventually, I stopped adding oil altogether. When dinner was ready, I made my mom put the rice on my plate and press it together in her hands so that I could see it was the same amount of rice I would eat regularly. I kept following this routine until I was banned from the kitchen.

Ever since the sickness started, my mom and I both knew that I had to follow strict diets, but I found a loophole. During every meal, I asked my mom to make small exceptions. For example, when she would be serving my dinner, I would plead for a "concession." This meant that she would serve a little less rice or would put fewer pieces of chicken on my plate. Day in and day out, I would ask for concessions. I knew that if my mom said yes, I would be eating less. Of course, when I cried and pleaded, my mom couldn't say no, so I got a concession almost every time I asked for one.

10

SINGAPORE: TO DECIDE OR NOT TO DECIDE

It is common knowledge that men don't cry. Patriarchs are supposed to be the glue of the family, the strong leaders who don't let anything affect them. But I learned the hard way that this isn't always true.

We were coming back from Sydney after our first New Year's Eve living in Asia. It was a beautiful trip. We climbed the Harbor Bridge, kayaked on the bay, went to the zoo, and saw the iconic fireworks on New Year's Eve. Yes, we did have problems with the food, and yes, I did lose weight, but in my memory, that trip was one of the most beautiful I have ever experienced. However, something was bound to go wrong.

We were on the plane heading back to Singapore, and everything was fine—until dinner was served. Plane food is horrible. I know no other way to describe it. Everyone dreads the moment the plane attendant comes by your seat with a huge, fake smile and asks if you want the week-old fish or the chemically bonded chicken. Of course, I didn't want to eat either, partly because of the caloric intake. My mother and I started our routine of bargaining, and at the far end of our row, my dad was watching us, closely observing our interaction.

My mom and I were both crying, but we were no longer fighting. I covered myself with a blanket and sobbed, shaking like crazy. My anxiety was at its peak level, and now instead of only being in mental pain, I was in physical pain, too. I went to the back of the plane and entered the restroom, calming myself so as to not cause a scene, but when I got back to my seat, the world had just fallen apart. My mothers' tears were still dripping down her face like a poorly closed faucet, and my dad's tears were apparent as well.

As far back as I can remember, I had never seen my dad cry. In fact, none of us, my mother included, had ever seen my dad cry. I looked at him in a way I never had before. He had always been my superhero, the person I admired the most because of his humor, perseverance, and strength; now, he looked like a fragile, abandoned puppy. His face red, as if straining to hold back the tears, yet his emotions were pouring out once and for all. That is the thing with feelings; they are like bombs. You have to be very careful with them because if you don't dismantle the bomb correctly, it will explode, and that is what was happening to all of us.

My mother had never faced her insecurities. She had always been extremely hard on herself because she always wanted to please her family. That is why, when I was diagnosed with anorexia, depression, obsessive compulsive disorder, and anxiety, she was later diagnosed with depression. My father grew up in a household with a very strict father. Yes, his family was loving and he was happy, but because he thought that men weren't supposed to cry, he never did. When I was diagnosed, he was also diagnosed with anxiety a few months later. The bomb inside all of us had exploded, and our bodies collided into a mess of emotions.

I ran toward my dad, not knowing how to react. What should I do? What should I say? The roles were reversed, and the tables had turned. I sat on his lap and simply hugged him.

"It's going to be okay," I said. " I just got a little anxious, but it's okay."

He looked at me with a new look in his eyes. "Please don't fight with your mom," he said, looking toward her. She was still sobbing. I nodded and told him that my reactions were not always in my control, but that I would try my best to eat what I had to.

After that, during every meal, I repeated my new mantra: focus on what is important. Is it your family or your body shape? Is it your life or the thickness of your legs? Focus on what is important.

Nevertheless, I struggled with the voices. I listened to them sometimes and did what they told me to. After all, it is hard to win a battle when you don't have the weapons to fight.

IT'S ON ME

It had been almost two years of chronic sadness, two years of hearing voices inside my head, two years of physical and mental chaos. I had been going to personal psychologist sessions for about six months. I hated Wednesdays because I knew I had to go to that small office with only two chairs and one couch, the room where I was supposed to talk about feelings I didn't even understand. I was helpless and consumed by too many voices at one time: my mother's, my father's, my counselor's, my family's, and the demon's.

My parents had been trying to convince me to talk to a girl who had previously suffered from anorexia and recovered, but I was never going to open up. I didn't need her help. I could get over this on my own. I just knew there had to be a specific epiphany moment in which the voices would just go away, and all of this would be over.

Nevertheless, everything stayed the same, despite six monotonous months of counseling in Singapore and the previous counseling I received in Chile. Nothing got better, and I simply became exhausted, tired of everything. This feeling reached such a point that I couldn't get out of bed.

Again and again, my parents insisted I try a different counselor or at least text the girl who had recovered from an eating disorder, and I eventually gave in. My cousin gave me the girl's contact number. I tried writing different messages, but none of them actually expressed what I needed to say. I began one text, deleted it completely, and then started again, never having the courage to send either. I could not find the exact words to explain what I was going through. I didn't really know what to say or how to start the conversation.

One day, I simply couldn't take it anymore. I was consumed by darkness and horrible thoughts. If I really wanted this horrible roller coaster of emotions to end, I had to look for help. I wrote everything that came to mind, all my experiences and what I had been feeling, and sent the recovered girl a text.

She answered almost immediately. She wrote me back, telling me her story and how she had gotten through the anorexia. She reassured me that she also heard the nagging voices and that I wasn't going crazy. We corresponded for a while until I finally dared to ask her what to do to get better. It was such a simple question, yet the answer changed my life. The three words she wrote altered every thought inside of my head: "It's a decision."

I had always known that the eating disorder was not in my hands. The eating disorder was something entirely out of my control, but *the solution* was in my power. Recovery *was* my choice.

"It's your choice," she said. "Start trying to eat some of your fear foods at least once or twice a week. Try ice cream, pizza, bread . . . maybe even some vegetables alongside your food. It won't hurt you, and that's what you need to realize. I made my choice. I decided that I wasn't going to let the eating disorder consume me and keep me from living my life. I decided that I was going to see life as it really is: a miracle that should be enjoyed, not suffered."

I didn't know how to answer. During the next few weeks, I convinced myself I was making the correct decision in trying to eat more, yet every now and then, I would throw away a little rice. Even though I was so tired and thought I wanted to get better, I hadn't armed myself for battle. The evil voices kept getting the better of me.

Every morning, I ate two pieces of toast with ham, chocolate milk, and fruits. I would wake up early simply to be the one to put the bread in the toaster. The toaster had eight heat levels, and I would always use the sixth because the toast would burn and then I would have an excuse to scrape off part of the bread. Also, when one opens the bag of bread, there is one very thin slice of bread on the top and another one at the bottom. I would always save those pieces because, after all, there was less bread and, thus, fewer calories.

The same cycle continued until one day I let the voices drown me. I sat with tears glistening in my eyes and just listened.

You are not good enough.

You don't deserve your family.

You have to throw away food because they are giving you more than you need.

You should run away.

You cause so much suffering.

I took in every negative thought and just let it be. Shortly after, it was time for dinner, and this time, I didn't throw anything away.

I had managed to stop throwing food away, but I still counted everything I ate. Fifty-five goldfish, ten grapes, twenty-nine almonds, four strawberries, and if the numbers didn't match up, I would leave the remaining in the container. I would walk through the hallways counting every gram of food, feeling every calorie.

Even though I kept going to my therapy sessions every week, the exhausting cycle continued. In addition, every week my mother weighed me to see if my weight was stable. Since my anxiety didn't let me sleep, I woke up extremely early, and every Saturday, I would have to wait for my mom to make my breakfast and weigh me. I thought that if I held my pee, I would weigh more and then my mom would not give me as much food. Thus, I held my pee all throughout the morning until my mother weighed me. The message my new friend had texted me echoed in my head: it's a choice. I had to choose between sickness and health.

I thought I was making the correct choice, but what normal thirteen-year-old counts how many goldfish she is eating? How many people count the number of raspberries they ingest? Even though the eating disorder fought to stay in control, recovery was ultimately in my hands.

COMMANDEERING MY MIND

From the day I made the correct decision, that I would actually make an effort to get rid of the eating disorder, my life changed in a tiny way. When I was eating snacks, I could feel the Bludger in my head trying to force me to count. After all, if I didn't, I might get hurt.

Nevertheless, I repeated the mantra my father had always said: Be strong. Be happy. And, to stop counting the food, I started singing in my head. Either that or if I realized I was counting, I would blurt out random numbers as if to confuse my own brain. It was a mess, a total blur of interactions between my heart and my mind, but I was finally starting to control myself once again.

A few weeks passed, and abruptly, my counselor had to leave to go to her hometown because of a health issue. So, once again, I was left alone in the darkness to cope with the voices. My mother recommended my friend's counselor as she was the professional who actually helped her get out of the eating disorder, but I refused. I stubbornly declined, feeling anger all around me. *We don't even know this person,* I thought. *Why does my mom trust her so much if we haven't even spoken to her?*

Yet, one day, my mother simply handed me the phone, and there she was. Since the counselor was all the way over in Colombia, and there was a time difference, we had to Skype right before I was going to bed. As the call connected, I saw a woman on a couch with a dog on her lap and a horrible view of Bogota behind her.

"So, tell me," she said, "tell me about the voices. Tell me about everything."

And I did. I was as open as I could be. I had to do something because I couldn't manage the voices anymore. She listened attentively, nodding as I told her my story.

Suddenly, she interrupted and said, "You're drinking from a cup made by God but poisoned by the devil. Put your hands together in prayer and repeat after me: I'm sorry, Lord, that I wanted to take my life. I'm sorry for what I've done to my parents. I'm sorry for what I've done to myself. Forgive me, Lord, forgive me."

I had to repeat this many times. Fear crept into my veins. I felt tingles on my arms as if spiders were crawling on my skin, their little legs sinking into the tissue. It was something that I had never felt before. I started crying, bawling, as I never had, yet I repeated everything she said.

I had never been very religious and neither had my parents. We are not devoted Catholics who go to church every Sunday. And, I had always had my doubts about religion. If such a benevolent God exists, why does he impose such suffering on people who have done nothing wrong? Don't get me wrong. I am not atheist, but I simply do not believe in the conventional God pictured in the Bible. In spite of that, her prayer made me feel guilt and fear and sadness and anger, all at the same time. I thought, *Am I really drinking poison from the devil? What is going on?*

The counseling session continued for the next hour, and after it finished, I lay down in bed and started shaking. It was as if I had been bewitched. My breaths got shorter. I felt tears stream down my face, and I had the tired feeling one has before fainting. My parents stormed into the room and huddled close, my dad on my left and my mom on my right.

"Everything is going to be okay," my dad muttered, rocking me back and forth.

"What happened?" my mom asked, yet I didn't answer. I had lost my voice and the feeling in my legs as well.

"I can't talk to her again," I said, and I continued bawling. The night continued, the week continued, the month continued, and I still felt the never-ending chronic fear and sadness. It was evident that we needed to find another solution. That was when we started Family-Based Treatment.

Before coming to Singapore, my mother had made an appointment at the Better Life clinic, but they only treated adolescents, and since I wasn't thirteen, they couldn't help me. Now, since my birthday had passed, they could finally help us.

I first went to visit the psychiatrist. Since I had been seeing another doctor, who had helped me get rid of the medicines the crazy scientist in Chile gave me, all of my information had to be transferred from one clinic to the other, but my medication didn't change. For the first time in two years, a doctor gave us a document with a full diagnosis: anorexia nervosa, anxiety, depression, and obsessive compulsive symptoms.

The psychiatrist said that we had two treatment options. One was to do independent (traditional) therapy, meaning that I would keep going to a one-on-one counselor and nutritionist and things would basically stay the same. The other option was Family-Based Treatment (FBT), which "empowered parents." The parents and doctors would work together to help me gain weight, and we would all do therapy together; that is why it is called Family-Based Treatment. The doctor said that the most efficient method of recovery was FBT, but I obviously didn't like it because it meant gaining weight. As soon as we left the clinic, I started crying.

"Mom, we can't do the second option. I will have to gain weight, and you will have to be tough with me. I don't want that!"

"I know, Caro," she answered with tears in her eyes. "Don't worry. We are not going to do FBT. I'm not strong enough to do it, and your father travels too much." Tranquility ran over me. I wasn't going to have to gain weight!

A week passed, and my parents decided that, indeed, we would be doing Family-Based Therapy. My father would cancel all his trips, and we would do therapy as a family. After all, it was the most efficient method, and we had run out of options.

Fear took me over. I had no idea what was coming my way.

That same week, we went to a new psychiatrist and were sent to a new therapist, but this time, I wasn't going to therapy on my own, merely talking about my feelings. We were doing something as a family.

The group of doctors helping us seemed to fit the definition of superheroes. In my mind, I saw them concocting plans to fight evil; the only difference was that, unlike traditional superheroes, the evil was inside children's minds. Consenting to treatment at that seemingly inconspicuous clinic meant I was sent home and forced to start a fast-paced, weight-gaining diet.

It amazes me how such an innocent-looking clinic must have witnessed so much suffering. Many people had walked into those offices and never returned. Others lived through the torture of weight gain while fighting to survive. I was scared. After all, the therapist told me that 50 percent of children with anorexia died. They either killed themselves or starved. I was part of the other 50 percent (for now), but I was at the low end of the graph. I was at the eighteenth percentile for weight, which meant that of girls my age and height, only 18 percent had that certain weight or lower. For me, percentiles were always extremely confusing, but I did know I should be at 50 percent or higher. The doctor told me that if my weight lowered to the tenth percentile, I would have to be hospitalized because my heart would stop working.

Facts and numbers were thrown at me, but the thing that stuck with me was when doctor said, "You have to commit yourself to the process because I am not going to another wake. Frankly, I want to see you for the least possible time, and let's hope that at the end of the year you won't need to come again. This will only happen if you are dedicated."

The second FBT session was complete and utter torture. I had to leave school early because part of the treatment involved a "family lunch" in which my whole family would cram into a small room and eat lunch in front of the doctor. She wanted to see how I would react with food, and she wanted to give my parents tips on how to manage me.

I entered the room controlling my emotions. After many years of going to a psychologist, I knew that every single thing I did would be interpreted. I couldn't give the wrong impression, not with food.

My mom slowly pulled out the containers of food, and as she opened one of them, I saw fried chicken. *Fried chicken.* I had not eaten that dish in approximately two years. And now my mom was going to force me to eat it, in front of the therapist, just to prove how damaged I was?

As if the fried chicken wasn't enough, my mom also pulled out mashed potatoes. I saw dairy and carbohydrates all mixed into one mush of calories. Anger coursed through my veins, burning through my skin until I could feel a sizzling feeling through my whole body. My mom also served vegetables, something I had never eaten before, even prior to this whole eating disorder fiasco.

I looked at her with the most accurate definition of a death stare. I started rambling in Spanish, feeling hot tears course down my cheeks. For the first time, I did not know how to express myself in English, even though the therapist could only understand English. I withheld my screams by squeezing my father's hand.

"Calm her down," the therapist told my parents.

"No soy un perro!" I yelled, unable to control my rage.

"What does that mean?" the therapist asked, genuine curiosity on her face. I didn't answer her; I simply glared at my plate.

"She is saying she is not a dog," my mom finally said.

"You are treating me like a dog!" I yelled. "You are giving me commands and forcing me against my will. It wouldn't surprise me if you tell me to roll over or play dead and then force fried chicken down my throat."

"A dog would eat the fried chicken happily," the therapist responded, "as should you."

I wasn't going to let her win. I have never considered myself a stereotypical teenager, rebelling or acting tough, yelling at my parents for no reason. But this time, my rebellion was about finishing my food. I wasn't going to let her say that I wasn't working hard enough. I wasn't going to let the therapist smirk after I failed to complete the simple task of eating a meal. Hence I gulped everything down. I sat there, my feet restless and my eyes blank, thankful that the worst part had ended. Just as I thought we could leave, my mom pulled a box of Guylian chocolate out of her purse.

She did not just do that.

These chocolates had always been my favorite. I fought with my brother over the chocolate that was shaped like a seahorse every time my mom brought home one of those boxes, but this time it was different. I hadn't eaten any sort of treats for the past two years—unless I was forced to—and I definitely hadn't eaten chocolate.

My brother's face lit up as he shot his hand into the box and grabbed the seahorse, but my mom stopped him. She took the seahorse and placed it right in front of me. I broke. I started screaming and crying and dry heaving. All of the worst feelings in the world had just ambushed me and were kicking me in the gut.

"You just want to make me look weak in from of the therapist!" I yelled at my mom. "You just want me to be sick!" Her eyes watered, and my dad squeezed my wrist. He pulled me over onto his lap and stroked my hair.

"It's okay. It's going to be okay," he said. Okay? What a strange thing to say to someone going through such pain. *It will be okay.* I don't know what effect those words had on me, but I grabbed the chocolate and gulped it down in one bite, without even chewing. Everyone at the table started at me in shock, and the therapist shook her head.

"You did absolutely nothing there; it was like you didn't eat the chocolate," the therapist said, and as if there were some invisible cue between them, my mother grabbed another chocolate and put it in front of me.

"Enjoy it this time," my mom said. I couldn't help but scowl.

FAMILY-BASED TREATMENT

There are three phases to FBT. The first phase is to gain all the weight lost. I was tired. So tired. After all, I had already been sick two years, and I knew I couldn't keep living with the eating disorder. So, I gained weight quickly by consuming foods high in calories.

In the second phase, parents slowly give the child more control. In my case, my parents started letting me serve my own food or choose what time I would eat. At this point, the voices could still, at times, consume me; however, they were less present. One doctor told me that the voices were caused by a chemical imbalance in the brain. Losing so much weight caused some chemical in the brain to react aggressively, causing the voices. I wish I could explain this better, but I don't understand it well myself. This illness is, after all, very abstract. Once I gained weight, the voices slowly faded. They were still there, but they were softer.

The counselor I saw at the beginning of my stay in Singapore once described the eating disorder as a chair in the room. You enter the room, acknowledge its presence, and move on. Of course, this is a silly analogy, but because this illness is so complicated, simple and silly things tend to make processing information much easier.

The third phase of FBT is "recuperating all that was lost." For example, one could go out with friends without a parent guarding you, and you could go exercise with the confidence that you won't overdo it. This treatment is called Family-Based Treatment because everyone has a role to play. My mom was the one who would manage all of my food. This is something she had always done; however, because the eating disorder's manipulation, she would give me concessions. With the help of my dad, she would resist the eating disorder's coercion to give me less food. I say "the eating disorder" because it was not me who manipulated. I was not in control, no matter how guilty I felt. My brother's job was to distract me. He would talk to me while I was eating so that I wouldn't spiral and let anxiety overpower me. All of these elements combined to build our family's FBT experience.

We followed the orders by the book. As soon as we got home from that first appointment, my parents started packing me with food:

- ✓ Milkshakes.
- ✓ Peanut Butter.
- ✓ Ice cream.
- ✓ Ensure.
- ✓ Pastries.
- ✓ Chocolate.
- ✓ High-calorie bars.

Anything and everything that would get my weight up was on the list. It was a horrible feeling, having to drink a milkshake with apples and peanut butter after already having dinner, but it was the only way I could get out of this. I know that many people talk about wanting to gain healthy weight, and that was my mindset as well, but healthy weight is very subjective, and I didn't have the time to stop and think or breathe or blink. I had to eat.

In a week, I gained two kilos, and in a month, I gained ten kilograms. Finally, I was at my appropriate weight. I was out of the danger zone.

All of this went back to what my friend and fellow anorexia sufferer had told me: it's a decision. I decided to eat everything put in front of me. I decided to finish all of the ice cream in the bowl, knowing it was the *most healthy option* for me at the time because, if I didn't eat all of it, I could die, and I knew it.

SUMMER BODY

May went by in the blink of an eye. After suffering so much, I felt stronger. I saw myself in a different light. I could go back to eating regularly again. Nevertheless, vacations were coming, and the voices were still not completely gone. We hadn't seen our extended family in about a year and a half, so this was the ultimate test. We were going to go back home, and then we would stop at Amsterdam on our way back to Singapore. Then we'd tour around China and Japan. If I could survive this without throwing any food away, without bargaining and bickering, I knew that the war between me and the eating disorder would come to an end. That tree that had taken root in my mind and grown way too big was being cut down, slowly but surely.

Even so, we had to continue the weekly appointments with the therapist because, despite having reached a healthy weight, I was far from recovered. Because of the time differences, my dad, who had stayed back in Asia, had to wake up at five in the morning as our therapist had to be at work by ten, and my whole family had to remain awake until eleven to participate in family treatment sessions. It was as if we were trapezing through time zones to keep my therapy sessions on track. Obviously, none of us lasted long having to be awake at such weird hours, so we collectively decided that the therapy sessions could be every two weeks.

During that time, I was still gaining weight. I needed to gain two more kilos, which would be the buffer that was needed in case I started losing weight because of sickness or any other *normal* reasons. I started going to the movies, to dinners and lunches, every day getting out of my comfort zone a bit more. Of course, the voices were still there.

One day, I had finished eating my lunch and everything was normal, but that is the thing with demons; they come out when you least expect it. Suddenly everyone decided to go and get ice cream. I wasn't prepared for that. I had eaten meatballs (which are fried) and a few fried plantains, so I couldn't eat more fat. I just couldn't. I left the table in a hurry and ran into my room crying. My mom came in running after me.

Eating disorder thoughts consumed me, eating away at my tranquility. What would happen if I ate that ice cream? Would I get fat? What would happen if I didn't eat the ice cream? Would it matter either way? After going back and forth, I was able to calm down. Recovery was in my hands, and if I let the eating disorder consume me like this, I would never get out of the dark hole.

I composed myself and announced that we had to go buy the ice cream. After all, my grandma always said that if you scratch your car or crash it when learning to drive, you have to get into the driver's seat immediately; you can't let the fear keep you from driving again. And that is what I was going to do. The anxiety "crash" wasn't going to make me take steps backward. The only way to prove the eating disorder wasn't in control was to disobey it. Looking back, as hard as it is to say, I am proud of how I reacted at that moment. I believe that if I hadn't been strong, I would have never advanced again.

I continued having those anxiety attacks, but I didn't feel alone anymore. Once, I simply needed to cry, and not a minute passed before my cousin rushed to my side to comfort me. We stayed there, and she heard my sorrows. She stroked my hair and told me it was going to be okay. That was all I needed. I couldn't have asked for more.

CODE RED

After being in Colombia for a month, I had gotten to my ideal weight, and it was time to go back to Asia. Asia's food is very different from what I am used to and what I actually like. Asian food in China or Japan is very different from the Chinese food or sushi Westerners are used to. For example, in Japan, there are no California rolls. Food was complicated, but it was a wonderful trip as we made our way back to Singapore.

We visited Tokyo and Kyoto, Xi'an and Beijing, with our most memorable day being a sunny afternoon in Beijing. My mother, brother, and I went to a puppet painting class. We sat down and started painting our rice film dragons, coloring them with ink and appreciating the patience these artists must have to have to put on a whole show. Our hands were stained with the ink, so, as any reasonable person would do, we went to the bathroom to wash up. As I entered the bathroom, I remembered an April Fool's day, a few months before I got diagnosed, when I went to the bathroom and told my brother to scream, "Caro is bleeding!" My mom climbed the stairs nonchalantly, and when she saw me sitting on the toilet, she completely freaked.

"You got your period? Really?"

I smiled and showed her the toilet water. It was stained red all over but not with blood—with food coloring.

"Carolina! You scared me! You know periods don't look like that, right?" She wore an angry face, but when I smiled, she started laughing like crazy.

Ever since that day, my mother confessed that every time I called her from the bathroom (usually to get toilet paper), she would cross her fingers and let the little candle of hope shine bright, thinking that I had finally gotten my period.

Because I didn't have enough fat in my body after the weight loss, I had stopped developing (which I had started at the ripe age of nine). The real sign of physical recovery would be to get my period once again. Once one starts gaining rapid weight, the body enters hoarding mode. All the weight I was gaining went directly to my belly area because that is where the principal organs are. That fat eventually disperses throughout one's whole body, but the period was something one simply had to wait out.

So, that morning in Beijing, I went to the bathroom and headed into a stall. As soon as I sat down, I saw the deep red stain.

"Mooooom!" I yelled. She came running in, her eyes wide open in hope. I only had to nod and a smile covered her whole face.

"Mom, I think I have ovarian cancer. I don't think this is my period."

"Shut up," my mom responded. "I am going to get you a pad!" She said this last phrase as if it were the chorus of a song. The rest of the day, my mom loaded me up with tips and tricks. It was easy to see that she had been waiting for the day to tell me all of this.

I took my phone out to tell my mentor-friend about that little red stain. She was the one who had made me realize that the way out of the darkness was in my hands. Afterward, I texted all of my family and became overwhelmed by the beautiful responses of support and love. They understood that this was an integral part of my recovery.

One day when I was living in Chile, I remember sitting at the foot of my parents' bed, looking out the window and making a promise to myself: *the day I get better, I will remember this very moment, which is filled with immense pain.* The moment I got my period for the first time, I thought of that long-ago moment.

I could finally see the light.

11

SINGAPORE: STEP BY STEP, PIECE BY PIECE

Months passed, and I still suffered with anxiety and depression. We had to adjust my pills various times and even considered making me go weekly to a psychologist, but after having to go to a counselor every week since fourth grade, one can understand that I was too tired to do any of this. Even so, my life was coming back, piece by piece. I would still fret if I wanted ice cream, but I ate it anyway because I knew that it was merely the eating disorder trying to get inside my head again.

I was prohibited from going to health class at school, for they taught us how to read the food labels and count calories, something which is medically proven to increase the number of eating disorders in a community. The therapist I was going to always reminded us that those nutrition classes were a threat to the health of the students, but, of course, the school wouldn't listen when I tried to explain the downside of these courses.

One day I walked into science class without a care in the world, only to be surprised that we were creating a machine that would burn food so that we could figure out how many calories the food had. I knew that a project like this was coming, but I didn't expect it to be so soon. I had been working for a long time, trying not to focus on calories, trying to forget diet-culture's definition of fat that I had memorized.

My hands were sweating, and an earthquake started moving in my chest. The teacher brought out popcorn and marshmallows, yet he unwittingly also brought out my anxiety. Not knowing what to do, I left the classroom, saying I had to go to the bathroom. In reality, I was frantically calling my mom. My hands shook as I picked up the phone. I thought I was better. I thought a scenario like this wasn't going to trigger me as much as it did. I tried to explain the situation to my frantic mother, who could not believe the school was teaching us how to find calories.

For some inexplicable reason, my anxiety had heightened that week. My mother told me to go immediately to the counselor. It was like an FBI raid. The school counselor went into my science class and got all of the stuff I had left behind, and after talking to me, he told me to wait in the conference room. I stayed there, and the world continued. Nothing changed. Nothing happened. I wished that the world would stop and suffer with me sometimes. I think it is so strange how someone can be feeling so much pain while another person is having the time of their life. It is a selfish thought and abstract, but it's very real for me.

After a year of sitting alone in the cafeteria, surrounded by so many people yet feeling utterly alone, I was happy to find out that a girl moved from the United States to Singapore. She was from Venezuela, and our school counselor put us in contact before the school semester started so that I could help her adapt. In the back of my mind, I also knew that we were connected so that I could adapt as well. In some inexplicable turn of fate, our mothers had been introduced by common friends of a common friend.

This is one of the bewildering things about being a Latina. Everyone knows everyone, and that is why you should never mess with one of us. You do this, and you will have all of Latin America knocking at your door.

It is safe to say that our friendship was meant to be. One day, my newfound friends and I were in the cafeteria after lunch. Before going down the stairs that led to our classes, we had to wait until one girl finished eating her cinnamon roll while the other finished her strawberry drink. As many times before, we were talking about weight. More accurately, *they* were talking about weight. I don't quite remember how the conversation started, but I knew things were going south when they started talking about numbers.

Time and time again, I had told them that if they didn't gain weight from fatty foods, there was never going to be anything to turn into muscle. I said all of this knowing that I had once committed the same mistakes they were making. At the beginning of my anorexia, I wanted muscle, but I didn't want to eat. Thus, due to all the energy I was burning, my body started to eat its own muscles because there was no more fat to burn. Nevertheless, it seemed as if they built an ice wall against reason whenever the word "fat" was uttered; of course, I used to do it, too.

We were walking out of the cafeteria after eating lunch, and mind you, I was still trying to recover from anorexia.

"How much do you weigh?" one girl asked.

"Okay. Don't laugh at me or anything, but I weigh thirty-nine kilograms," my friend said.

"Wow," the other responded, "you are so light!"

"Yeah, I know. It's not my fault that I am a small, anorexic little girl. Have you seen my arms? I can't even lift weights!"

"Wait," the other responded. "Are you anorexic?"

"No!" she answered. "What do you think?"

"Did you know I was anorexic once? Hey, Caro, how much do you weigh?"

Oh, no. My turn.

Why was this important? Yes, I had seen both of my friends look at themselves in the mirror, exclaiming their dire necessity for abs. Everything came to a point when one of them stood sideways in front of me with her shirt up, showing me how her belly looked when she was squeezing it in versus how it looked when she was not. All of these girls and boys, consumed with thinking about their weight and appearance, their belly, their abs, their arms—all things I used to worry about. Yet, I took them to a deadly extreme.

"I don't think that it is important," I answered. Looking back, I wish I would have told them my weight. I wish I hadn't been such a coward. What was the problem with weighing fifty-one kilograms, thirty-four kilograms, or one hundred kilograms? Yet, I let my insecurities get the better of me.

Perhaps one of the most difficult things about anorexia has been dealing with the ignorance and misconceptions surrounding the disorder and the current conceptions regarding weight, body image, and self-esteem. When I finally told my best friend about my disease, she was thunderstruck. She was going to health class, but I could not. We had become such close friends that it pained me to lie to her about why, so I simply blurted out my situation.

"I need to tell you something, but please don't freak out. I don't want this to change the way you see me."

She froze in her tracks and looked at me with surprise. "Is it bad?" she asked.

"Kinda"

"Don't tell me," she responded. "I don't want to know, then."

"Ok," I said, legitimately surprised. I had prepared a whole dramatic dialogue in my head, and she simply did not want to know the "bad thing" going on in my life. *What exactly does that mean?*

"Never mind," she decided, "tell me."

"Okay, well, I suffered from anorexia for two years. I'm still in recovery, and health class is a huge trigger. That is why I can't go."

Her already huge eyes widened as if she had seen the devil himself. It was the first time I had opened up to someone about anorexia. I was able to tell her how much it enraged me when the other girl claimed she was anorexic and that the only thing she talked about was calories. Point number one, you can't *be* anorexic; you are not the sickness. You can *suffer* from anorexia, and it is important to distinguish these two phrases. Point number two, I couldn't handle the constant blabber about calories. I used to do that, and I ended up at the lowest and darkest place of my life. To this day, I still do not go to health class because I am afraid that if I hear the teachers rant about calories it will wake up the monster within me.

As you may notice, people today are becoming more and more obsessed with food and calories. Yes, one should try to be as healthy as possible, but to decline something that makes you happy because you know that it has calories? The worst part of it is that thousands of kids and adults who have recovered have to suffer through ignorance and misconceptions, all of which can be a trigger to pull them—us—down.

Sometimes people act as if they are divine beings who are omniscient and all-knowing, as if they are the keepers of diet truths, and no one can tell them otherwise. Even people in my very household have had to change their mindset because of my eating disorder.

Another great difficulty has been learning to conquer my fear of food. Although things have gotten so much better, I am still afraid of food and very conscious about the small part of my brain that tells me to eat less. Anxiety springs on me when my routine is broken.

One day, a friend gave me and my other friend a brownie. Of course, my friend ate the brownie, but my head was spinning with indecisiveness. Should I eat it? If I do, do I eat my afternoon snack? Do I eat a lighter dinner? After all, I hadn't eaten a brownie in more than two years. I had no idea what the repercussions were going to be, but that was exactly what pushed me to eat it. I ate half of the brownie and immediately called my mom because anxiety was attacking me. But it was okay. That one brownie was going to do absolutely nothing to my weight, and it would show my eating disorder that it doesn't control me, not anymore. I ended up eating the other half of the brownie as well and my afternoon snack, and I lived to tell the story.

During the last few months, I have relearned what it feels like to crave food and feel hungry, even after a hearty meal. But most importantly, I have relearned what it feels like to be happy and guilt free. Food is what keeps me alive. I chose to live and continue fighting, and now it has paid off.

Nevertheless, I am still struggling with depression and anxiety. My psychiatrist once told me that going into anorexia was like walking through a tunnel. The walls were all experiences, thoughts, and moments that built what was the eating disorder. Now that I am getting better, it is as if I am walking backwards through the same tunnel, reliving many emotions similar to the ones I felt when all of this started. The difference is that now I have a choice. I can continue pulling myself down and eventually relapse, or I can face my fears and stand up to the bully in my head to get out of this tunnel once and for all.

I graduated from FBT on January 17, 2019. I am still medicated for anxiety and depression, and we may even have to increase my dosage because the depression is still a powerful part of my life. However, my life is so much better. I am happy most of the time. I can laugh and joke around, just like before.

Ever since I can remember, I've begged my parents for a dog, but my mom always found an excuse to say no. It was because we lived in an apartment or because I wasn't ready, but one night, I decided to take matters into my own hands. While my parents were out with friends, I stayed home and researched. I knew I wanted a pug, so I just had to find one and coordinate everything so that my mom had no reason to say no.

After hours of looking online, I found the perfect breeder. Without consulting my parents, I contacted the man with the pug, and he sent me a picture of a small, fragile black pug. It is safe to say that I fell in love. Once my parents came home, I had already figured out the price and all of the arrangements to make this puppy ours. After so much pain, after so much suffering and grasping the thin thread that is life, I just wanted a clumsy puppy to make me laugh. I believe that we all needed the dog.

A week later, my parents and I made our way to the breeder and adopted Nala, the weirdest pug in the world. I look at her and want to laugh, and every time I laugh, I remember that I once couldn't bear to smile. Nala has a huge tongue that doesn't fit in her mouth, floppy ears that bounce when she runs, and an incredible ability to make me happy.

One day, my brother, my father, and I all went to Sentosa in Singapore to do an activity together. We were attached to this huge trampoline that allowed us to jump extremely high. The first few jumps made my stomach churn and my head dizzy, but once I got used to it, I felt as if I could reach the stars. I did forward flips and backward flips, and my brother did the same. Seeing how much fun we were having, my dad decided to join in. They strapped him onto the trampoline, and he attempted to do a forward flip. Everything went in slow motion as he got stuck in mid-air, just when he was about to hit the trampoline again. His head was where his legs were supposed to be as his neck hit the trampoline.

I heard a huge scream of pain. I looked at my brother and then at my dad, who had finally disentangled himself, rubbing his neck, and I erupted into laughter. I laughed and laughed and laughed. Suddenly, my dad and brother laughed as well. My stomach started aching, and I even peed myself a little. After I finally caught my breath, I realized I hadn't laughed so much in more than two years. At that moment, I realized my happiness was slowly coming back. My *life* was coming back.

I have no certain rules about what I should or shouldn't eat at this stage. I eat what I want, and at this point, my parents trust me enough—I trust myself enough—to rest knowing that I am making decisions about what I eat and how much I exercise based on sound reason—not a distorted voice in my head. Nevertheless, I am still going to my psychiatrist every few months so that she can monitor my weight and my emotional progress. It is estimated that I have to do this for another year to be sure I am back on track.

I know the eating disorder will always be with me. I know I will have to live with a part of this eating disorder forever. I know there is a possibility of relapsing, but realizing this is precisely what keeps me from going into the dark hole once again. I understand this is a mental issue and that mental health is a power often out of one's control, just like cancer or ALS. As a survivor, I understand this disorder is not my fault, that I am not my eating disorder. I am merely the victim of a hurricane.

Many pains have come with this illness, but I have grown in immeasurable amounts. My family has become so much closer due to our ability to express our emotions with more freedom. Negative judgment toward others has been eradicated, and our minds are more open and accepting. In addition, we are all on a journey to be happy with ourselves. It is not only me who has had to improve self-esteem. With my mom's depression and my dad's anxiety, we are all learning to embrace ourselves.

I don't want this to be a sad story or one that people will pity. For me, this was and will always be a learning experience. The tree is still growing, but the roots are healing and will eventually let healthy leaves flourish.

I have learned that I am stronger than I ever thought I could be. I've learned that I deserve happiness and love and that it is never acceptable to deprive myself of vital necessities, such as food and joy. After all this time, I have indeed learned that even in the direst of circumstances, there is an upside of being down.

ABOUT THE AUTHOR

Speaking three languages, living in five countries, and organizing a successful annual fundraiser, Carolina Mejia Rodriguez wrote her first book as a thirteen-year-old. In addition to winning school awards ranging from the Scholastic Art and Writing Award to the President's Award of Academic excellence, Carolina is a member of the National Junior Honors Society. As a third-culture-kid, Carolina has been able to raise money from around the world for a group of children in need in Colombia called Las Estrellas del Rawad. Carolina has been featured on the daytime Emmy-award-winning show *Despierta America,* creating consciousness about Anorexia Nervosa in teenagers.